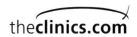

UROLOGIC CLINICS
OF NORTH AMERICA

Contemporary Issues and
Management of Bladder Cancer

GUEST EDITOR
John P. Stein, MD, FACS

CONSULTING EDITOR
Martin I. Resnick, MD

May 2005 • Volume 32 • Number 2

SAUNDERS

An Imprint of Elsevier, Inc.
PHILADELPHIA   LONDON   TORONTO   MONTREAL   SYDNEY   TOKYO

W.B. SAUNDERS COMPANY

A Division of Elsevier Inc.

1600 John F. Kennedy Boulevard • Suite 1800 • Philadelphia, Pennsylvania 19103-2899

http://www.theclinics.com

THE UROLOGIC CLINICS OF NORTH AMERICA
May 2005
Editor: Catherine Bewick

Volume 32, Number 2
ISSN 0094-0143
ISBN 1-4160-2801-3

The ideas and opinions expressed in *The Urologic Clinics of North America* do not necessarily reflect those of the Publisher. The Publisher does not assume any responsibility for any injury and/or damage to persons or property arising out of or related to any use of the material contained in this periodical. The reader is advised to check the appropriate medical literature and the product information currently provided by the manufacturer of each drug to be administered to verify the dosage, the method and duration of administration, or contraindications. It is the responsibility of the treating physician or other health care professional, relying on independent experience and knowledge of the patient, to determine drug dosages and the best treatment for the patient. Mention of any product in this issue should not be construed as endorsement by the contributors, editors, or the Publisher of the product or manufacturers' claims.

The Urologic Clinics of North America (ISSN 0094-0143) is published quarterly by W.B. Saunders Company. Corporate and editorial offices: Elsevier, Inc., 1600 John F. Kennedy Blvd., Suite 1800, Philadelphia, PA 19103-2899. Accounting and circulation offices: 6277 Sea Harbor Drive, Orlando, FL 32887-4800. Periodicals postage paid at Orlando, FL 32862, and additional mailing offices. Subscription prices are $195.00 per year (US individuals), $307.00 per year (US institutions), $225.00 per year (Canadian individuals), $371.00 per year (Canadian institutions), $260.00 per year (foreign individuals), and $371.00 per year (foreign institutions). Foreign air speed delivery is included in all *Clinics* subscription prices. All prices are subject to change without notice. POSTMASTER: Send address changes to *The Urologic Clinics of North America*, W.B. Saunders Company, Periodicals Fulfillment, Orlando, FL 32887-4800. **Customer Service: 1-800-654-2452 (US). From outside the US, call 1-407-345-4000.**

The Urologic Clinics of North America is covered in *Index Medicus, Excerpta Medica, Current Contents/ Clinical Medicine, Science Citation Index,* and *ISI/BIOMED.*

Printed in the United States of America.

CONSULTING EDITOR

MARTIN I. RESNICK, MD, Lester Persky Professor and Chairman, Department of Urology, Case Western Reserve University, School of Medicine/University Hospitals, Cleveland, Ohio

GUEST EDITOR

JOHN P. STEIN, MD, FACS, Associate Professor of Urology, Department of Urology, Norris Comprehensive Cancer Center, University of Southern California Keck School of Medicine, Los Angeles, California

CONTRIBUTORS

LIANA ADAM, MD, PhD, Assistant Professor, Department of Urology, The University of Texas M.D. Anderson Cancer Center, Houston, Texas

ANA M. APARICIO, MD, Assistant Professor of Medicine, Division of Medical Oncology and Kenneth J. Norris Comprehensive Cancer Center, University of Southern California Keck School of Medicine, Los Angeles, California

FIONA C. BURKHARD, MD, Department of Urology, University of Bern, Bern, Switzerland

SAM S. CHANG, MD, Assistant Professor, Department of Urologic Surgery, Vanderbilt University Medical Center, Nashville, Tennessee

PETER E. CLARK, MD, Assistant Professor of Urology, Wake Forest University Health Sciences, Winston-Salem, North Carolina

MICHAEL S. COOKSON, MD, Associate Professor, Department of Urologic Surgery, Vanderbilt University Medical Center, Nashville, Tennessee

COLIN P.N. DINNEY, MD, Professor and Chairman, Department of Urology, The University of Texas M.D. Anderson Cancer Center, Houston, Texas

ANTHONY B. ELKHOUIERY, MD, Assistant Professor of Medicine, Division of Medical Oncology and Kenneth J. Norris Comprehensive Cancer Center, University of Southern California Keck School of Medicine, Los Angeles, California

M. CRAIG HALL, MD, Professor of Urology, Wake Forest University Health Sciences, Winston-Salem, North Carolina

RICHARD E. HAUTMANN, MD, Professor of Urology and Chairman, Department of Urology, University of Ulm, Ulm, Germany

HARRY W. HERR, MD, Department of Urology, Sidney Kimmel Center for Prostate and Urologic Cancers, Memorial Sloan-Kettering Cancer Center, New York, New York

WASSIM KASSOUF, MD, Fellow, Department of Urology, The University of Texas M.D. Anderson Cancer Center, Houston, Texas

THOMAS M. KESSLER, MD, Department of Urology, University of Bern, Bern, Switzerland

S. BRUCE MALKOWICZ, MD, Professor, Division of Urology, Department of Surgery, University of Pennsylvania School of Medicine and the Abramson Cancer Center of the University of Pennsylvania, Philadelphia, Pennsylvania

MURUGESAN MANOHARAN, MD, FRCS(Eng), FRACS(Urol), Assistant Professor, Department of Urology, University of Miami School of Medicine, Miami, Florida

MICHAEL A. O'DONNELL, MD, Associate Professor and Director of Urologic Oncology, Department of Urology, University of Iowa College of Medicine, Iowa City, Iowa

DAVID F. PENSON, MD, MPH, Departments of Urology and Preventative Medicine, University of Southern California Keck School of Medicine, Los Angeles, California

MICHAEL P. PORTER, MD, MSE, Department of Urology, University of Washington, Seattle, Washington

DAVID I. QUINN, MD, PhD, Assistant Professor of Medicine and Director, Clinical Investigations Support Office, Division of Medical Oncology and Kenneth J. Norris Comprehensive Cancer Center, University of Southern California Keck School of Medicine, Los Angeles, California

DONALD G. SKINNER, MD, Department of Urology, Norris Comprehensive Cancer Center, University of Southern California Keck School of Medicine, Los Angeles, California

MARK S. SOLOWAY, MD, Professor and Chairman, Department of Urology, University of Miami School of Medicine, Miami, Florida

JOHN P. STEIN, MD, FACS, Associate Professor of Urology, Department of Urology, Norris Comprehensive Cancer Center, University of Southern California Keck School of Medicine, Los Angeles, California

URS E. STUDER, MD, Department of Urology, University of Bern, Bern, Switzerland

DAVID J. VAUGHN, MD, Associate Professor, Division of Hematology/Oncology, Department of Medicine, University of Pennsylvania School of Medicine and the Abramson Cancer Center of the University of Pennsylvania, Philadelphia, Pennsylvania

JOHN T. WEI, MD, MSE, Department of Urology, University of Michigan, Ann Arbor, Michigan

CONTENTS

**Practical Applications of Intravesical Chemotherapy and Immunotherapy
in High-risk Patients with Superficial Bladder Cancer**   121
Michael A. O'Donnell

> With recurrence rates after transurethral surgery commonly exceeding 60%, adjuvant intravesical therapy should be considered for all intermediate- and high-risk patients with superficial bladder cancer. Immediate one-dose perioperative cytotoxic chemotherapy should be applied whenever feasible. For intermediate-risk patients, a full induction cycle of chemotherapy or bacillus Calmette-Guérin (BCG) immunotherapy is appropriate. Further maintenance therapy is helpful in select patients. For high-risk patients, BCG is preferred along with at least a year of maintenance therapy. Failures with high-risk disease may require cystectomy, but salvage programs using BCG plus interferon or gemcitabine can provide additional clinical responses for patients with lower-risk recurrences or those medically unfit or refusing aggressive surgery.

Optimal Management of the T1G3 Bladder Cancer   133
Murugesan Manoharan and Mark S. Soloway

> Management decisions for a patient with a high-grade T1 urothelial cancer of the bladder are both critical and controversial. The optimal management of these tumors requires an accurate diagnosis including the stage and grade, and careful assessment of prognostic factors. The wide range of available treatment options includes transurethral resection alone, adding intravesical therapy, radical cystectomy, and even possibly chemoradiation. Despite advances in the understanding of the biologic behavior of these tumors, both the choice and timing of treatment remain controversial.

Radical Cystectomy for Bladder Cancer: The Case for Early Intervention 147
Sam S. Chang and Michael S. Cookson

> For practicing urologists, determining the timing for radical cystectomy can be difficult. In the absence of clinically proven biomarkers for predicting tumor biology and the response to therapy, the decision needs to be tailored for each patient. Unfortunately, for many patients, the window of opportunity may be shorter than expected, and recent studies have demonstrated the negative effect of a delay in cystectomy. This article reviews the indications and proposed benefits of proceeding expeditiously with radical cystectomy.

removal of the bladder. As urologists have become more experienced with different forms of urinary diversion, perioperative complication rates have become comparable, as have cancer control and overall survival. For these reasons, health-related quality of life (HRQOL) outcomes are an important component in assessing therapy for invasive bladder cancer. This review discusses measurement of HRQOL in bladder cancer patients who require cystectomy, reviews the current studies examining HRQOL in these patients, and describes approaches that will allow future studies to address this important issue more accurately.

Urothelial transitional cell cancer has a high rate of response to combination cytotoxic therapy. Approximately 50% of patients with high-grade bladder cancer and deep muscle invasion ultimately die of disseminated disease. Translating the high response seen in locally advanced disease into long-term survival in the metastatic setting and to improved survival in the advanced setting has proved difficult. This article reviews the use of adjuvant chemotherapy in localized or locally advanced transitional cell cancer. The chemotherapy of urological malignancies, including bladder cancer, has recently been reviewed in detail; this article does not contain an extensive review of the drugs used.

Muscle-invasive bladder cancer is a highly lethal disease. Radical cystectomy and bilateral pelvic lymph node dissection can have a significant impact on survival, but outcomes are determined by pathologic stage. Many patients with extravesical or lymph node positive bladder cancer will develop recurrent disease—often with distant metastases—and will ultimately die from their disease. Given the lethality of muscle-invasive bladder cancer, there is a definite need for effective systemic chemotherapy. This article examines the role of neoadjuvant chemotherapy in muscle-invasive bladder cancer.

The tremendous amount of data accumulated through genomics, proteomics, and metabolomic technologies has not led to a definitive understanding of the mechanisms underlying cancer. The challenge remains as to how to integrate all of the relevant knowledge and data in a systematic manner so that researchers can gain the knowledge needed to devise the best therapeutic and diagnostic strategies. Human transitional cell carcinoma of the bladder is genetically heterogeneous, and it is surrounded by a complex tissue microenvironment involving vasculature, stromal cells, and connective tissue. One of the most challenging problems facing cancer researchers is the lack of correlation between in vitro cell lines and animal tumor models and human in vivo tumors. A few promising approaches are being devised that will help address this issue in the coming years. One such approach is the measurements of molecular levels of receptors, ligands, pathways components, and so on, directly in human tumors through in vivo imaging, or through proteomic profiling, as it has been proposed as standard protocol for cancer diagnostics and therapeutics.

GOAL STATEMENT

The goal of *Urologic Clinics of North America* is to keep practicing urologists and urology residents up to date with current clinical practice in urology by providing timely articles reviewing the state of the art in patient care.

ACCREDITATION

The *Urologic Clinics of North America* is planned and implemented in accordance with the Essential Areas and Policies of the Accreditation Council for Continuing Medical Education (ACCME) through the joint sponsorship of the University Of Virginia School Of Medicine and Elsevier. The University Of Virginia School of Medicine is accredited by the ACCME to provide continuing medical education for physicians.

The University of Virginia School of Medicine designates this educational activity for a maximum of 60 category 1 credits per year, 15 category 1 credits per issue, toward the AMA Physician's Recognition Award. Each physician should claim only those credits that he/she actually spent in the activity.

The American Medical Association has determined that physicians not licensed in the US who participate in this CME activity are eligible for AMA PRA category 1 credit.

Category 1 credit can be earned by reading the text material, taking the CME examination online at http://www.theclinics.com/home/cme, and completing the evaluation. After taking the test, you will be required to review any and all incorrect answers. Following completion of the test and evaluation, your credit will be awarded and you may print your certificate.

FACULTY DISCLOSURE

As a provider accredited by the Accreditation Council for Continuing Medical Education (ACCME), the Office of Continuing Medical Education of the University of Virginia School of Medicine must ensure balance, independence, objectivity, and scientific rigor in all its individually sponsored or jointly sponsored educational activities. All authors/editors participating in a sponsored activity are expected to disclose to the readers any significant financial interest or other relationship (1) with the manufacturer(s) of any commercial product(s) and/or provider(s) of commercial services discussed in an educational presentation and (2) with any commercial supporters of the activity (significant financial interest or other relationship can include such things as grants or research support, employee, consultant, stock holder, member of speakers bureau, etc.) The intent of this disclosure is not to prevent authors/editors with a significant financial or other relationship from writing an article, but rather to provide readers with information on which they can make their own judgments. It remains for the readers to determine whether the author's/editor's interest or relationships may influence the article with regard to exposition or conclusion.

The authors/editors listed below have identified no professional or financial affiliations related to their presentation:
Liana Adam, MD, PhD; Ana Aparicio, MD; Catherine Bewick, Acquisitions Editor; Fiona C. Burkhard, MD; Sam S. Chang, MD; Michael Cookson, MD; Colin P. N. Dinney, MD; Anthony B. Elkhouiery, MD; M. Craig, Hall, MD; Harry W. Herr, MD; Wassim Kassouf, MD; Thomas M. Kessler, MD; S. Bruce Malkowicz, MD; Murugesan Manoharan, MD, FRCS; David F. Penson, MD, MPH; Michael P. Porter, MD, MSE; Martin I. Resnick, MD, Consulting Editor; Donald G. Skinner, MD; Mark S. Soloway, MD; John P. Stein, MD; Urs E. Studer, MD; David J. Vaughn, MD; and, John T. Wei, MD, MSE.

The authors/editors listed below have identified the following professional or financial affiliations related to their article:
Michael O'Donnell, MD is a consultant and has received grant funding from Schering and rEli Lilly; he is also a consultant for Medical Enterprises, Sanofi-Aventis-Pasteur-Merieuxt.
David Ian Quinn, MD is on the speakers' bureau for Aventis, Merck, OSI, Millennium, Abbott, Cytogen, MGIPharm, Chiron and has received research support from Millennium and Aventis.

Disclosure of Discussion of non-FDA approved uses for pharmaceutical products and/or medical devices: The University of Virginia School of Medicine, as an ACCME provider, requires that all faculty presenters identify and disclose any "off label" uses for pharmaceutical and medical device products. The University of Virginia School of Medicine recommends that each physician fully review all the available data on new products or procedures prior to instituting them with patients.

The following authors who provided disclosure will be discussing the off-label use of the following pharmaceutical or medical device products:
Ana Aparicio, MD, Anthony B. Elkhouiery, MD, and David Ian Quinn, MD will discuss the use of paclitaxel, docetaxel, and all drugs listed in table 5 of their article.
Michael O'Donnell, MD will dicuss the use of Interferon- alpha, gemcitabine, and microwave hyperthermia for treatment of superficial bladder cancer.
Donald G. Skinner, MD will discuss tntervesical chemotherapy for bladder cancer.

The authors/editors listed below have not provided disclosure or off-label information:
Elizabeth Louise Bahn, MD, PS; Peter E. Clark, MD; and, Richard E. Hautmann, MD.

TO ENROLL

To enroll in the Urologic Clinics of North America Continuing Medical Education program, call customer service at 1-800-654-2452 or visit us online at www.theclinics.com/home/cme. The CME program is available to subscribers for an additional fee of $165.00

FORTHCOMING ISSUES

RECENT ISSUES

THE CLINICS ARE NOW AVAILABLE ONLINE!

Access your subscription at:
http://www.theclinics.com

UROLOGIC
CLINICS
of North America

Urol Clin N Am 32 (2005) xi

Foreword

Contemporary Issues and Management of Bladder Cancer

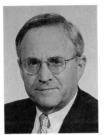

Martin I. Resnick, MD
Consulting Editor

Cancer of the bladder is the second most common malignancy of the genitourinary tract. Recent statistics from the American Cancer Society indicate that approximately 274,000 individuals will be diagnosed with the disease worldwide, and less than half (108,000) will succumb to it. Although in the United States the majority of patients have transitional cell carcinoma, in other regions squamous cell malignancies predominate. Traditionally, the only management available to these patients was surgical removal of the malignancy and if invasive extirpation of the bladder is necessary with associated urinary diversion. Many advances over the past decade have permitted more focused therapy resulting not only in eradication of the tumor but also preservation of the urinary bladder and its function.

Dr. John Stein, Guest Editor of this issue of the *Urologic Clinics of North America*, has compiled a monograph consisting of important and controversial topics written by experts in the field and has appropriately addressed traditional concepts in treatment as well as new approaches under development. Intravesical therapy and cystectomy and the role of chemotherapy and radiation therapy are reviewed, as are the important issue of quality of life and new surgical procedures that have been developed in neobladder construction that have benefitted this patient population.

All physicians who care for patients who have carcinoma of the bladder will find this issue of value. The topics presented are timely, the authors are well-recognized, experienced clinicians, and developments and innovation that have evolved are clearly presented.

Martin I. Resnick, MD
Lester Persky Professor and Chairman
Department of Urology
Case Western Reserve University
School of Medicine/University Hospitals
11100 Euclid Avenue
Cleveland, OH 44106-5046, USA

E-mail address: mir@po.cwru.edu

ELSEVIER
SAUNDERS

Urol Clin N Am 32 (2005) xiii–xiv

**UROLOGIC
CLINICS
of North America**

Preface

Contemporary Issues and Management of Bladder Cancer

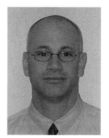

John P. Stein, MD, FACS
Guest Editor

The treatment of bladder cancer has evolved on various fronts over the past 20 to 30 years. Significant advances and discoveries in cellular biology and a better understanding of the molecular events and pathogenesis of this urologic malignancy have allowed clinical scientists to develop and study novel mechanisms in prevention and detection with innovative treatment plans for this disease. For this potentially morbid and lethal tumor, the improvements in the clinical and histopatholgic understanding of the disease are equally important and clearly more practical for the practicing physician, because they allow for improvements in risk assessment and treatment decisions. In addition, advances in the medical and surgical treatment of both superficial and invasive bladder tumors have occurred, allowing for better oncologic outcomes while attempting to maintain certain quality of life issues. Lastly, I believe future treatment of all malignancies may evolve toward a more target-based strategy with the use of small molecules in specific fashion.

An attempt has been made to address these clinical concepts in bladder cancer. This particular issue of the *Urologic Clinics of North America* was strategically developed around what I believe are important and contemporary clinical issues and dilemmas that confront the practicing urologist on a daily basis regarding bladder cancer. I hope the experience, expertise, and wisdom of the contributing authors will provide insight and elucidate some of these clinical predicaments. The goal is to provide the readership with a better understanding of the disease and to emphasize the various improvements in the overall treatment of the disease—ultimately so the patient with bladder cancer may benefit from better clinical and treatment decisions.

I am gratefully indebted to the authors who have contributed to this issue. It should be noted that the authors have been purposefully selected and include individuals who have dedicated themselves and their careers to the better understanding and treatment of patients who have bladder cancer. Their thoughtful expertise, insight, and experience with the disease have improved the care and clinical outcomes of those with the disease. Furthermore, I hope the overall contributions of these authors will provide the platform for younger and enthusiastic clinical scientists to continue to improve upon our better understanding and management of this tumor.

doi:10.1016/j.ucl.2005.03.003

urologic.theclinics.com

It has been a privilege to be the Guest Editor for this issue. I would like to thank all the families who have supported the authors (including my wife Randi and my children)—not only for their contribution to this endeavor, but also for their personal sacrifices that have been made to better understand and treat patients with bladder cancer. Finally, I would like to acknowledge Catherine Bewick, whose expertise and persistence made this project not only possible, but pleasant.

John P. Stein, MD, FACS
Associate Professor of Urology
Department of Urology
Norris Comprehensive Cancer Center
University of Southern California
Keck School of Medicine
1441 Eastlake Avenue, Suite 7416
Los Angeles, CA 90089-9178, USA

E-mail address: stein@usc.edu

ELSEVIER
SAUNDERS

Urol Clin N Am 32 (2005) 121–131

UROLOGIC
CLINICS
of North America

Practical Applications of Intravesical Chemotherapy and Immunotherapy in High-risk Patients with Superficial Bladder Cancer

Michael A. O'Donnell, MD

Department of Urology, University of Iowa College of Medicine, Iowa City, IA 52242-1009, USA

With the exception of first time, solitary, small-to-moderate sized, low-grade, stage Ta papillary bladder cancers, all other cases of superficial bladder cancer carry at least a 60% to 80% chance of 5-year recurrence following surgical ablation alone [1]. With these disappointing statistics, it is not surprising that adjuvant therapies have been developed in an attempt to reduce this high tumor recurrence rate. Aside from the risk for recurrence, in tumors with high-grade features, invasion into the lamina propria (stage T1), or carcinoma in situ (CIS), there is an even more pressing concern about progression to muscle invasion with its attendant life-threatening implications. For these high-risk patients, intravesical chemotherapy or immunotherapy is strongly recommended, even at the time of first presentation.

Initial steps: adequate resection and perioperative cytotoxic chemotherapy

Chemotherapy and immunotherapy have the capacity to ablate small (<1.5 cm) residual tumors; however, recurrence rates are never as good as when therapy is applied in the prophylactic (no visible disease remaining) setting [2]. It is mandatory that as complete a resection as possible be performed before starting intravesical therapy. In some cases, this may mean additional sessions to remove tumor completely and achieve adequate staging information. With bulky or multifocal high-risk tumors, studies have shown a 30% to 40% residual tumor rate and a similar

E-mail address: michael-odonnell@uiowa.edu

rate of understaging, especially if underlying muscle is not included [3,4]. Muscle invasive disease is not susceptible to topical agents; therefore, a failure to make this diagnosis virtually guarantees failure. CIS poses a different problem. Although in a minority of cases it may present as a focal region, most cases are diffuse and multifocal. Aside from adequate sampling, complete ablation is seldom recommended or even possible.

Based on more than two decades of clinical investigation recently recompiled in the form of a meta-analysis, there is overwhelming support for the use of one-dose immediate postoperative cytotoxic chemotherapy after transurethral resection (TUR) [5]. Although more commonly used for low-risk patients, in whom at a median follow-up of 3.4 years there is an approximate 39% drop in the odds of recurrence (ie, from 47% to 36% actual change in recurrence rate), the results for patients with multiple tumors are even better. These patients experience a 56% reduction in the odds of recurrence (ie, from 81.5% to 65%). With the exception of thiotepa, all of the cytotoxic agents studied (epirubicin, pirarubicin, mitomycin) seem equally effective. The relative noneffectiveness of thiotepa from the reviewed trial has been linked to the dilute strength used (30 mg in 50 mL) and the fact that up to 24 hours could have elapsed before drug administration [6]. Experience with mitomycin C has indicated that initiation of therapy within 6 hours is substantially more effective than after 24 hours [7]. The usual dwell time for the intravesical drug given perioperatively has ranged from 30 to 60 minutes. One study found that systemic absorption of mitomycin was no different for a 30- or 60-minute dwell time [8], whereas another found 60

Box 1. Strategies to erect an intravesical peri-operative chemotherapy plan

1. Meet with appropriate personnel (OR nursing, Pharmacy, Scheduling) to discuss medical need and logistical plans.
2. Include immediate peri-operative chemotherapy on actual operative schedule to alert staff.
3. Call pharmacy before or early into case to verify need for drug. This will minimize drug wastage. Note: certain drugs such as mitomycin are stable for 1 week at room temperature and 2 weeks refrigerated.
4. Try to cluster similar TUR bladder cancer cases together to maximize pharmacy efficiency.
5. Set up a closed system to minimize nursing contact with chemotherapeutic agent. For instance, place a 3-way catheter in OR attached to irrigant fluid (e.g., 1 liter normal saline) but turned off. Doctor administers the chemotherapy agent through the main catheter port, clamps with hemostat and attaches to drainage bag (system now closed). At agreed upon time (e.g., 60 minutes) have staff release clamp to drain drug into bag. Thereafter run 1 liter of saline through irrigant port over next 30–60 minutes. If satisfied with results, remove foley and discard along with urinary drainage bag into biohazard container. All staff should wear gloves.

---

minutes to be more effective [9]. Neither of these studies specifically investigated immediate perioperative dosing. Suspected perforations, large tumor bed resections, or continued moderate bleeding may justify a shorter exposure time, longer delay, or omission of this treatment altogether.

Generally, good tolerance has been observed with all of the agents given in the one-dose perioperative format. The choice of agent should be guided by personal experience and consideration of individual circumstances. Thiotepa is more easily absorbed than the other drugs such that up to one-half of the dose may become systemic. Mitomycin can cause a severe reactive cystitis or skin rash in a small percentage (approximately 5%) of cases. It also may leave a calcified eschar at sites of large resection, fortunately with little clinical consequence. Doxorubicin (Adriamycin) is the least expensive of current agents but is no longer widely used owing to reduced efficacy with long-term use. Although Adriamycin has been replaced by other anthracycline derivatives, such as epirubicin, there is disagreement about whether this is clearly advantageous. One comparative trial found reduced toxicity and suggested greater efficacy for epirubicin, whereas two other studies found no significant difference [10–12]. One-time perioperative use of doxorubicin may still be the most cost-effective option. Conventional immunotherapy should not be given perioperatively. Interferon-alpha (IFN-α) is ineffective, and bacillus Calmette-Guérin (BCG) can cause life-threatening sepsis in this setting [13,14].

Despite the fact that perioperative intravesical chemotherapy has proven efficacy after almost every TUR, it is not yet fully used in clinical practice (4% use in 1999 in a United States survey by author). The reasons for this are multiple and include unfamiliarity with evidence; concern about toxicity; cost and reimbursement, especially of unused drug; logistic delivery of drug to the surgical suite; and fear of chemotherapy drug exposure by medical staff. A practical methodology for institution of a perioperative program is provided in Box 1.

Choosing a post–transurethral resection regimen for previously untreated patients

Although one-dose perioperative chemotherapy is a vital first step in decreasing tumor recurrence, fully two thirds of patients with multifocal tumors will still relapse. A sequential regimen of repetitive intravesical therapy can provide additional benefit. The choice of whether this should be a chemotherapy- or immunotherapy-based program is determined not only by personal preference but also by a careful assessment of the risk-benefit ratio for the agent in a particular patient. Chemotherapy regimens are generally better tolerated than BCG and do not engender the real but small fear of severe BCG infections that occur in approximately 5% of patients [14]. Prior chemotherapy failure does not adversely affect the subsequent response to BCG. Furthermore, for patients with intermediate-risk features, such as multifocal or multirecurrent, low-to-intermediate grade, papillary Ta tumors, the chance of progression is rarely greater than 2% per year [1]. On balance, intravesical chemotherapy may be the most reasonable first step in these patients to achieve tumor control without risking toxic side effects. Indeed, most national consensus panels agree that intravesical chemotherapy is a worthwhile initial option for intermediate-risk groups [15,16].

The details of start time, the interval between doses, cycle length, dose, and dwell time have largely been established empirically and are relatively uniform for all chemotherapeutic drugs. Nevertheless, recent studies suggest that further optimization is possible. Treatment with chemotherapy can begin at any time postoperatively, although most clinicians wait 1 to 3 weeks. A minimum of four sequential treatments has demonstrated efficacy with mitomycin, but 6- or 8-week regimens are the most common. Up to 12 weekly treatments have been advocated by some, usually with a 2-week spacing between treatments in the latter half. Longer regimens are more commonly associated with greater degrees of chemical cystitis. Intolerance (dropout) rates range from 2% to 16% (Table 1). The drug dose (total amount) may not be as important as the actual concentration, because the latter determines the transit and depth of drug penetration across the bladder mucosa [17]. Although theoretically a longer drug dwell time should translate to heightened efficacy, dwell times beyond 2 hours have not been shown to be substantially better. Although part of this is due to practical limits of

bladder-holding volume, substantial drug dilution (often, fivefold to tenfold) over 2 hours destroys the concentration gradient [18].

Optimization of the delivery of intravesical chemotherapy has unequivocally demonstrated better clinical results in tumor recurrence rates for mitomycin. By eliminating the residual volume (confirmed by bladder scan), overnight fasting, increasing the mitomycin C (MMC) concentration to 40 mg in 20 mL, and achieving urinary pH alkalinization using oral bicarbonate to reduce MMC degradation, a doubling of the durable tumor-free rate was obtained in a randomized clinical trial [19]. Other practical methods to reduce ongoing drug dilution include a single 200-µg oral dose of desmopressin given 1 hour before treatment and temporary abstinence from caffeine or other diuretics [20]. Patients who have irritative bladders or reduced bladder capacity that prevents at least a 1-hour drug retention may similarly benefit from pretreatment with bladder antispasmodics and oral narcotics. It is likely that many of these optimization methods will also enhance the efficacy of other intravesical therapeutics with the exception of urinary alkalinization, which is unique to mitomycin. Increasing the total drug dose beyond the recommended range will not necessarily improve clinical outcome and may only increase local toxicity, as has been demonstrated in a study of intravesical epirubicin [21].

All conventional cytotoxic agents (thiotepa, mitomycin, the anthracyclines) induce cystitis to a varying degree (Table 1). There are also certain drug-dependent side effects [22]. Repetitive

Table 1
Comparisons between intravesical agents

Agent	MW	Peri-op Use	Risk Group	Cystitis %	Other Toxicity	Dropout %	Concentration	Cost*
Adriamycin	580	Yes	Low-Interm	20–40%	Fever, allergy ∼5%	2–16%	50 mg/50 cc	$36
Epirubicin	580	Yes	Low-Interm	10–30%	Contracted bladder rare	3–6%	50 mg/50 cc	$595
Thiotepa	189	Yes	Low-Interm	10–30%	Myelo-suppression 8–19%	2–11%	30 mg/30 cc	$80
Mitomycin	334	Yes	Low-Interm	30–40%	Rash 8–19% contracted bladder 5%	2–14%	40 mg/20–40 cc	$130
BCG	N/A	No	Interm-High	60–80%	5% serious infection	5–10%	1 vial/50 cc	$150
Interferon	∼23,000	No	Salvage	<5%	Flu-like Sx 20%	Rare	50–100 MU/50 cc	$670–$1340
Gemcitabine	300	Yes	Salvage	mild	Occasional nausea	<10%	1–2 gm/50–100 cc	$540–$1080

* Based on 2005 discount acquisition costs from oncology supply distributors.

dosing of thiotepa may cause serious myelosup-pression. Mitomycin induces an idiosyncratic hypersensitivity response in approximately 10% of patients leading to a genital palmar hand rash and (rarely) severe intractable cystitis. Anthracy-clines are associated with a somewhat higher incidence of irritative bladder symptoms, includ-ing urgency, pain, hematuria, and incontinence. In the United States, the unit cost for 40 mg of mitomycin is only slightly greater than that for 30 mg of thiotepa, whereas 50 mg of Adriamycin is roughly one-half to one-third the cost.

Maintenance chemotherapy

The use of additional treatments of intravesical chemotherapy after completion of the induction cycle at a time when the patient is already in complete clinical remission is known as "mainte-nance" therapy. The rationale for maintenance therapy is to prevent the emergence of new cancers from a diseased premalignant urothelium or to eradicate small clinically undetectable nests of residual cancer. The most common regimen involves monthly therapy, usually for at least a year, but variations of quarterly treatments, sequential miniseries, and more extended sched-ules also have been described.

Currently, the use of maintenance chemother-apy is controversial, with some studies showing benefit and others no benefit. Several early pro-spective clinical trials showed that an extended (1 year or more) maintenance program of doxo-rubicin or mitomycin was not superior to an induction regimen only [23–26]. In contrast, a higher efficacy was reported for long-term instillation of epirubicin versus short-term instil-lation [27]. In this prospective randomized trial, the patients received their first treatment within 24 hours, followed by epirubicin for 3 months or 12 months. The 3-year recurrence rate was 36% in the first group versus 15% in the second. Conrad et al [28] similarly found that 3 years of monthly MMC maintenance was superior to no mainte-nance (recurrence rate of 14% versus 31%) in patients with Ta G2/3 and T1 G1-3 tumors at a median follow-up of 2.9 years. In a meta-analysis of 11 randomized trials, Huncharek et al [29] suggested that chemotherapy for 2 years had the greatest effect on decreasing the recurrence rate.

Some clarification in resolving the mainten-ance chemotherapy controversy is provided by a European trial [30]. A combined analysis of two prospective randomized trials compared early (the day of resection) versus delayed (7 to 15 days after resection) and short-term (6 months) versus long-term (12 months) treatment with MMC or doxo-rubicin. Although no significant difference was reported in the disease-free interval among all groups, the recurrence rate was worse among patients who started treatment late and received no maintenance. This difference was supported by the findings in a randomized trial of early in-stillation of epirubicin with maintenance versus no maintenance, showing no difference in recurrence. Long-term maintenance chemotherapy is proba-bly unnecessary if perioperative chemotherapy is given in addition to the usual induction course; however, maintenance should be considered if perioperative chemotherapy has not been applied.

Intravesical immunotherapy

Based on an absolute superiority in activity coupled with an increased familiarity and accep-tance of its side effects, BCG has become the most popular choice for intravesical therapy in North America by an almost 2:1 majority. Interestingly, Europeans do not share this enthusiasm for BCG and use it only about one-third of the time. For low-to-intermediate risk cases of superficial blad-der cancer, primary chemotherapy and BCG re-main appropriate options; however, for high-risk cases, there is rather compelling evidence that first-line therapy should begin with BCG, single-dose perioperative chemotherapy notwithstanding.

In overall activity against papillary disease, BCG is about twice as effective as chemotherapy in preventing recurrence after TUR, providing an approximately 30% absolute advantage versus chemotherapy's 15% advantage over TUR alone [31]. In cases of CIS, BCG boasts more than a 70% complete response rate, whereas the results of chemotherapy are usually around 50% [32]. Most head-to-head comparisons between BCG and chemotherapeutic drugs have also favored BCG, with the exception of some mitomycin trials enrolling lower-risk patients. A recent set of meta-analyses of such comparative trials yielded the following important insights: (1) the relative ben-efit of BCG is greatest for high-risk groups [33]; (2) the best results for BCG are obtained when it is used for at least a year of maintenance therapy [33,34]; and (3) BCG is especially more effective in cases of prior chemotherapy failure [35].

More importantly, BCG has achieved dominance in the issue of prevention of tumor progression. Two separate meta-analyses have reached the same conclusion that BCG reduces the risk of progression. In one study, progression at 2.5 years' median follow-up was reduced by 27% (9.8% for BCG versus 13.8% for non-BCG) [36]. In another study, the reduction at 26-month median follow-up was 23% (7.7% for BCG versus 9.4% for MMC) [37]. Interestingly, in both cases, the superior results with BCG were only seen in trials using BCG maintenance therapy. No chemotherapy trials have ever shown a reduction in progression. Nevertheless, proof of a survival advantage associated with BCG remains lacking, largely encumbered by the low relative death rate for superficial bladder cancer and the need for very long-term clinical studies.

Optimized administration of bacillus Calmette-Guérin

As is true for intravesical chemotherapy, many details of BCG administration have not been subjected to scientific rigor; rather, they have been derived from empiric observations. At least 7 to 14 days should elapse after the TUR before beginning BCG. Earlier administration has been associated with BCG sepsis. Many clinicians choose to wait 3 to 4 weeks or longer until all postoperative bleeding is over. A full induction cycle usually consists of six weekly treatments, but 8- and 12-week schedules have also been reported. Simultaneous percutaneous BCG inoculation has proved to be of no benefit [38]. The usual dwell time is 2 hours. Methods to decrease early voiding as described previously for chemotherapy may be worthwhile.

No particular commercial strain or preparation of BCG has shown consistent clinical superiority; however, adequate BCG viability measured in terms of colony-forming units (CFUs) is required for optimal activity [39]. One full dose (one ampule or vial) varies in weight from strain to strain, but absolute CFUs remain similar. Several European studies suggest the BCG dose can be reduced safely to one-half to one-quarter a vial with a twofold to threefold reduction in toxicity while maintaining comparable efficacy [40–42]; however, the results seem to be better for the standard BCG dose in patients with multifocal tumors and high-grade disease [43]. Furthermore, given the widespread exposure

or inoculation of older Europeans to tuberculosis and BCG, it may not be possible to translate these findings directly to immunologically naive North American patients. Indeed, in the only study comparing reduced-dose BCG (60 mg Pasteur) with full-dose (120 mg Pasteur) BCG in North America, lower doses were associated with a significant reduction in activity (67% disease-free rate with the full dose versus a 37% rate with one-half dose) [44]. For North American patients known to have Tb/BCG exposure or prior BCG treatment, a dose reduction may be justified to enhance compliance, especially during re-induction or maintenance cycles.

Although various BCG regimens exist, the most effective programs have at least two aspects in common: (1) they allow a re-induction cycle for nonprogressing patients at first failure, and (2) they provide at least a year of maintenance therapy. Given the aforementioned results of several meta-analyses demonstrating the necessity of maintenance therapy to achieve superiority for reducing recurrence and progression, there is little doubt that a maintenance plan should be adopted, especially in higher-risk patients. The two most popular maintenance plans involve monthly therapy, or a series of 3-week minicycles at 3 and 6 months followed by repeat cycles every 6 months to 3 years. Although randomized studies using quarterly or monthly single treatments did not demonstrate a consistent benefit [45,46], the miniseries maintenance regimen was clearly superior to nonmaintenance in a randomized controlled trial by the Southwest Oncology Group (SWOG 8507 protocol) [47]. Of 233 randomized patients with CIS, 84% ultimately achieved a complete response with maintenance therapy versus 68% without. Of 254 patients with completely resected papillary disease and no recurrence at 3 months, 87% were disease-free at 2 years in the maintenance arm compared with 57% without maintenance. At least a 20% absolute differential persisted for up to 5 years. In the combined CIS plus papillary groups, the median recurrence-free survival was roughly doubled from 36 to 77 months. Even disease worsening was improved in the maintenance group by a statistically significant 6% differential. Nevertheless, one quarter of patients receiving maintenance therapy experienced significant grade 3 toxicity, and less than half completed more than three cycles, with only 16% completing all seven planned cycles. Because the maintenance group as a whole benefited even without most patients completing a full 3 years of therapy, the maximum benefit may have been achieved earlier. These results have been reproduced in two smaller studies in France and Poland [48,49]. In the French study, only 19% of patients completed the entire 3-year maintenance schedule. Conversely, a large European study found a 20% toxicity-related dropout rate [50]. Furthermore, nearly two thirds of all dropouts occurred during the first 6 months, suggesting that measures to reduce early toxicity are needed. A reduced BCG dose or slow dosing of BCG (every 2 weeks rather than weekly) may be beneficial in reducing dropout in patients showing signs of intolerance [51].

What to do when treatment fails

Despite the strides made with intravesical chemotherapy and immunotherapy, most patients will eventually have a recurrence of disease. For intermediate-and high-risk patients treated with chemotherapy, the answer is simple—try BCG next. For BCG failures, the problem is more complicated, because salvage chemotherapy with traditional agents rarely achieves a greater than 20% 3-year disease-free rate [52]. Because a second course of BCG still provides between a 30% to 50% response, it is probably worthwhile to consider this step for most initial BCG failures [53,54]. The exceptions would include patients worsening despite BCG and those with very high-risk conditions, such as multifocal stage T1G3 tumor with associated CIS. Because 3- to 5-year progression rates of 30% to 50% have been documented in such cases, immediate cystectomy may be the safest option [55,56]. Further courses of BCG beyond two are not recommended, because the durable response is usually under 20%, and the risk of progression escalates rapidly [57]. Nevertheless, other salvage programs may be appropriate for patients intolerant to conventional therapy, patients with less serious recurrence, patients unfit for cystectomy, or patients refusing cystectomy even after being properly informed of their risks.

Salvage programs

Role of interferon, alone and combined with bacillus Calmette-Guérin

Interferons are natural glycoproteins that mediate host immune responses such as the stimulation of phagocytes, cytokine release, enhanced natural killer cell activity, and activation of T and B lymphocytes. Of all the interferons, IFN-α has been the best studied as an intravesical treatment agent [58]. When used by itself, IFN-α is well tolerated, causing minimal cystitis and only occasional low-grade fevers or flulike symptoms [59]. Its efficacy is clearly dose dependent, with minimal activity at doses at or less than 10 million units (MU) and best activity at or above 50 MU. Moderate ($\geq$40%) dose-dependent clinical activity against papillary stage Ta bladder cancer in post-TUR (prophylactic) and in marker lesion (ablative) settings has been reported [60,61], but poor results are seen for stage T1 tumors [62]. Direct comparative studies have revealed that IFN-α is less effective as primary therapy than cytotoxic chemotherapeutics and BCG [61,63]. For this reason and its higher expense, its use has predominantly been restricted to salvage situations. For patients with CIS failing BCG, the complete response rate to IFN-α is approximately 15% to 20% at 1 year, with a durable response of approximately 12% by 2 to 3 years [64].

Combining IFN-α with BCG has been proposed as a viable option for BCG failures. Small single institution studies using low-dose BCG plus 50 to100 MU of IFN-α have demonstrated 1- to 2-year success rates of 50% to 60%, with better results with a second re-induction option and three sets of 3-week miniseries maintenance treatments 3, 9, and 15 months later [65–67]. The interim results of a large national multicenter phase II trial of combination BCG plus IFN-α in BCG naïve and BCG failure patients reveal similar findings [68]. BCG naïve patients (n = 259) received standard dose BCG plus 50 MU of IFN-α followed by three 3-week maintenance cycles with reduced dose BCG, whereas BCG failure patients (n = 231) were treated similarly with the exception of a reduced BCG dose plus 50 MU of IFN-α beginning at induction. Based on one induction cycle only, the Kaplan-Meier estimates for freedom from disease at 2 years were 57% for BCG naïve patients and 42% for BCG failure patients. There was minimal serious toxicity and a high level of patient tolerance, with less than 10% patient dropout owing to toxicity. Progression was seen in approximately 8% of both groups, implying that the BCG failure patients were not disproportionately disadvantaged. These encouraging results have led some to consider using combination therapy even as upfront therapy for primary bladder cancers; however, the incremental value of IFN in this setting has not yet been established.

New intravesical chemotherapy drugs

Given the generally poor results of conventional intravesical chemotherapy for BCG failures, new drugs have been sought to remedy this deficiency. Valrubicin, an anthracycline with a mechanism of action different from the parent compound Adriamycin, was approved by the Food and Drug Administration on the basis of a phase II study involving 90 patients with CIS after failure of multiple courses of intravesical therapy, including at least one course of BCG. After receiving 800 mg of valrubicin weekly for 6 weeks, 19 patients (21%) had a complete response at 6 months, and 7 of these 19 patients (8% of total) had a durable response with a median follow-up of 30 months [69]. Most patients (90%) had mild-to-moderate local bladder symptoms, with urinary frequency in 66%, urinary urgency in 63%, and dysuria in 60%. Unfortunately, the clinical availability of valrubicin has been severely curtailed.

Gemcitabine and the taxanes paclitaxel and docetaxel have demonstrated clear single agent activity against metastatic bladder cancer [70]. Early laboratory studies suggest that the taxanes can be formulated into an active intravesical treatment, but clinical studies have not yet been reported [71]. By contrast, multiple phase I and phase II trials of intravesical gemcitabine have been performed [72–74]. Usually formulated as 1 to 2 g in 50 to 100 mL of water or saline (final concentration, 20–40 mg/mL), gemcitabine can be safely administered either weekly or twice weekly for six to eight treatments. Minimal systemic absorption occurs through the bladder, and hematologic toxicity is rare. Transient nausea is the most common side effect. Chemical cystitis is generally mild.

Objective activity has been demonstrated for gemcitabine in multiple settings. In 9 of 13 evaluable patients receiving gemcitabine for prior failure of treatment for papillary disease, no recurrence was seen at 3-month follow-up [72]. The chemoablative activity of intravesical gemcitabine was recently reported in a marker lesion study in patients with papillary Ta T1 grade 1 to 2 disease [75]. In a sample size of 39 patients, 2 g of gemcitabine in 50 mL of saline given weekly for 6 weeks was able to ablate 56% of the marker lesions completely. Particularly relevant for salvage therapy is the report by Dalbagni et al using a twice per week program for 3 weeks, followed by a second cycle after a week of rest, in a heavily pretreated population with BCG-refractory transitional cell carcinoma, mostly CIS. A complete response, defined by a negative posttreatment cystoscopy, biopsy, and cytology, was achieved in 7 of 18 patients (39%) in a phase I study [73]. This study was followed by a phase II investigation in a further sample of 28 patients with BCG-refractory transitional cell carcinoma, of whom 16 (57%) achieved a complete response [76]. All of the aforementioned reports suffer from a lack of long-term data to measure response durability. The feasibility of a sequential gemcitabine-mitomycin regimen has been reported by O'Donnell et al [77], with 70% success in 10 heavily pretreated patients at 9-month median follow-up.

Emerging technologies

Although not yet readily available to urologic practitioners in North America, two device technologies developed in Europe that facilitate drug delivery are showing great promise for primary and salvage therapy. Local hyperthermia using a specially designed microwave antennae Foley catheter in conjunction with concomitant MMC therapy (chemothermotherapy) has demonstrated encouraging results in ablating large tumor burdens as well as preventing recurrence after TUR of bladder tumor [78,79]. Randomized trials comparing chemothermotherapy versus intravesical mitomycin alone have shown large differences in the recurrence rate (17% versus 57% at 24 months). This modality has been applied to patients with high-grade superficial bladder cancer (Ta T1 G3), with a 62.5% recurrence-free rate in the prophylactic group after a mean follow-up of 35.3 months and 75% ablation (total recurrence-free rate of 80.9%) at a mean follow-up of 20 months [80]. Early reports have also documented success in prior BCG or chemotherapy failures [81].

Electromotive intravesical MMC therapy (eMMC) provides yet another method to boost chemotherapy tissue penetration and anticancer efficacy. Di Stasi et al [82] randomized three groups of patients with CIS to 40 mg of eMMC instillation with 20 mA of electric current for 30 minutes, 40 mg of passive MMC with a dwell time of 60 minutes, or 81 mg of BCG with a dwell time of 120 minutes. Patients were scheduled for an initial six weekly treatments, a further six weekly treatments for nonresponders, and a follow-up ten monthly treatments for responders. There was a statistically significant superior complete response rate at 6 months for eMMC (58%) when compared with passive MMC (31%). The response rate of eMMC approached that of BCG (64%). Peak plasma MMC was significantly higher following eMMC than after passive MMC (43 vs 8 ng/mL), supporting the hypothesis that eMMC increases tissue levels.

Photodynamic therapy, previously falling out of favor owing to local and cutaneous toxicity from using photofrin, may be set to re-emerge with better technology and photosensitizing intravesical agents. Photodynamic therapy after oral administration of 5-aminolevulinic acid (ALA) was performed in 24 patients with recurrent superficial transitional cell carcinoma after BCG [83]. At a median follow-up of 36 months, three of five patients with CIS and 4 of 19 with papillary transitional cell carcinoma were free of disease. In another study using intravesical ALA in 31 patients with superficial bladder cancer, 10 of whom had a recurrence of disease after BCG therapy, 16 were recurrence free at an average follow-up of 23.7 months, whereas 15 patients had a recurrence after a mean of 8.3 months. Of ten patients with prior BCG treatment, four (40%) were free of tumor recurrence [84]. Therapy was well tolerated; minimal side effects included dysuria and hematuria. A new intravesical sensitizing agent being tested, hypericin, may be even more favorable than ALA [85]; however, as is true for all of these emerging technologies, treatment is still restricted to a small number of centers, usually in the context of clinical trials.

Summary

The following steps are practical in the treatment of intermediate-to-high risk patients with superficial bladder cancer:

Resect all visible tumor at the time of first TUR of bladder tumor. Strongly consider re-resection, especially for high-risk, large, multifocal, stage T1 tumors.

Apply one dose of cytotoxic chemotherapy perioperatively within 6 hours of TUR (ideally immediately).

Once histopathology is available, consider intravesical induction chemotherapy for intermediate-risk patients and BCG for intermediate- or high-risk patients and those having failed prior chemotherapy.

At least 1 year of maintenance therapy should be planned for all intermediate-to-high risk

BCG-treated patients. Chemotherapy maintenance may be useful if perioperative chemotherapy was omitted.

For patients failing standard therapy, a thorough discussion of the risks (including progression and metastasis) and expected benefits should take place before the initiation of salvage therapy. The radical cystectomy option should be openly entertained.

Consider BCG plus interferon or gemcitabine-based salvage programs if appropriate. Explore clinical trial options. Contact urologic cancer experts for guidance and advice.

References

[1] Millan-Rodriguez F, Chechile-Toniolo G, Salvador-Bayarri J, et al. Primary superficial bladder cancer risk groups according to progression, mortality and recurrence. J Urol 2000;164:680–4.

[2] Maffezzini M, Simonato A, Zanon M, et al. Up-front intravesical chemotherapy for low stage, low grade recurrent bladder cancer. J Urol 1996;155: 91–3.

[3] Klan R, Loy V, Huland H. Residual tumor discovered in routine second transurethral resection in patients with stage T1 transitional cell carcinoma of the bladder. J Urol 1991;146:316–8.

[4] Herr HW. The value of a second transurethral resection in evaluating patients with bladder tumors. J Urol 1999;162:74–6.

[5] Sylvester RJ, Oosterlinck W, van der Meijden AP. A single immediate postoperative instillation of chemotherapy decreases the risk of recurrence in patients with stage Ta T1 bladder cancer: a meta-analysis of published results of randomized clinical trials. J Urol 2004;171:2186–90.

[6] Medical Research Council Working Party on Urological Cancer, Subgroup on Superficial Bladder Cancer. The effect of intravesical thiotepa on tumour recurrence after endoscopic treatment of newly diagnosed superficial bladder cancer: a further report with long-term follow-up of a Medical Research Council randomized trial. Br J Urol 1994;73:632–8.

[7] Kaasinen E, Rintala E, Hellstrom P, et al. FinnBladder Group: factors explaining recurrence in patients undergoing chemoimmunotherapy regimens for frequently recurring superficial bladder carcinoma. Eur Urol 2002;42:167–74.

[8] van Helsdingen PJ, Rikken CH, Sleeboom HP, et al. Mitomycin C resorption following repeated intravesical instillations using different instillation times. Urol Int 1988;43:42–6.

[9] Giesbers AA, Van Helsdingen PJ, Kramer AE. Recurrence of superficial bladder carcinoma after intravesical instillation of mitomycin-C: comparison of exposure times. Br J Urol 1989;63:176–9.

THERAPY FOR SUPERFICIAL BLADDER CANCER

[10] Shuin T, Kubota Y, Noguchi S, et al. A phase II study of prophylactic intravesical chemotherapy with 4'-epirubicin in recurrent superficial bladder cancer: comparison of 4'-epirubicin and adriamycin. Cancer Chemother Pharmacol 1994;35(Suppl): S52–6.

[11] Eto H, Oka Y, Ueno K, et al. Comparison of the prophylactic usefulness of epirubicin and doxorubicin in the treatment of superficial bladder cancer by intravesical instillation: a multicenter randomized trial. Kobe University Urological Oncology Group. Cancer Chemother Pharmacol 1994;35(Suppl): S46–51.

[12] Rajala P, Kaasinen E, Raitanen M, et al. Finnbladder Group. Perioperative single dose instillation of epirubicin or interferon-alpha after transurethral resection for the prophylaxis of primary superficial bladder cancer recurrence: a prospective randomized multicenter study—FinnBladder III long-term results. J Urol 2002;168:981–5.

[13] Ali-el-Dein B, el-Baz M, Aly AN, et al. Intravesical epirubicin versus doxorubicin for superficial bladder tumors (stages pTa and pT1): a randomized prospective study. J Urol 1997;158:68–73.

[14] Lamm DL. Complications of bacillus Calmette-Guerin immunotherapy. Urol Clin North Am 1992;19:565–72.

[15] Oosterlinck W, Lobel B, Jakse G, et al. European Association of Urology (EAU) Working Group on Oncological Urology: guidelines on bladder cancer. Eur Urol 2002;41:105–12.

[16] Smith JA Jr, Labasky RF, Cockett AT, et al. Bladder cancer clinical guidelines panel summary report on the management of nonmuscle invasive bladder cancer (stages Ta, T1 and TIS): the American Urological Association. J Urol 1999;162:1697–701.

[17] Kuroda M, Niijima T, Kotake T, et al. Effect of prophylactic treatment with intravesical epirubicin on recurrence of superficial bladder cancer—the 6th Trial of the Japanese Urological Cancer Research Group (JUCRG): a randomized trial of intravesical epirubicin at dose of 20 mg/40 mL, 30 mg/40 mL, 40 mg/40 mL. Eur Urol 2004;45:600–5.

[18] Chai M, Wientjes MG, Badalament RA, et al. Pharmacokinetics of intravesical doxorubicin in superficial bladder cancer patients. J Urol 1994; 152:374–8.

[19] Au JL, Badalament RA, Wientjes MG, et al. International Mitomycin C Consortium. Methods to improve efficacy of intravesical mitomycin C: results of a randomized phase III trial. J Natl Cancer Inst 2001;93:597–604.

[20] Cliff AM, Heatherwick B, Scoble J, et al. The effect of fasting or desmopressin before treatment on the concentration of mitomycin C during intravesical administration. BJU Int 2000;86:644–7.

[21] Masters JR, Popert RJ, Thompson PM, et al. Intravesical chemotherapy with epirubicin: a dose response study. J Urol 1999;161(5):1490–3.

[22] Thrasher JB, Crawford ED. Complications of intravesical chemotherapy. Urol Clin North Am 1992;19: 529–39.

[23] Flamm J. Long-term versus short-term doxorubicin hydrochloride instillation after transurethral resection of superficial bladder cancer. Eur Urol 1990; 17:119–24.

[24] Rubben H, Lutzeyer W, Fischer N, et al. Natural history and treatment of low and high risk superficial bladder tumors. J Urol 1988;139:283–5.

[25] Huland H, Kloppel G, Feddersen I, et al. Comparison of different schedules of cytostatic intravesical instillations in patients with superficial bladder carcinoma: final evaluation of a prospective multicenter study with 419 patients. J Urol 1990;144: 68–71.

[26] Akaza H, Isaka S, Koiso K, et al. Comparative analysis of short-term and long-term prophylactic intravesical chemotherapy of superficial bladder cancer: prospective, randomized, controlled studies of the Japanese Urological Cancer Research Group. Cancer Chemother Pharmacol 1987;20(Suppl):S91–6.

[27] Koga H, Kuroiwa K, Yamaguchi A, et al. A randomized controlled trial of short-term versus long-term prophylactic intravesical instillation chemotherapy for recurrence after transurethral resection of Ta/T1 transitional cell carcinoma of the bladder. J Urol 2004;171:153–7.

[28] Conrad S, Friedrich MG, Schwaibold H, et al. Long term prophylaxis with mitomycin C (MMC) further reduces tumor recurrence compared to short term prophylaxis with MMC or bacillus Calmette-Guerin (BCG). J Urol 2004;171:71A.

[29] Huncharek M, Geschwind JF, Witherspoon B, et al. Intravesical chemotherapy prophylaxis in primary superficial bladder cancer: a meta-analysis of 3703 patients from 11 randomized trials. J Clin Epidemiol 2000;53:676–80.

[30] Bouffioux C, Kurth KH, Bono A, et al. Intravesical adjuvant chemotherapy for superficial transitional cell bladder carcinoma: results of 2 European Organization for Research and Treatment of Cancer randomized trials with mitomycin C and doxorubicin comparing early versus delayed instillations and short-term versus long-term treatment. European Organization for Research and Treatment of Cancer Genitourinary Group. J Urol 1995;153:934–41.

[31] O'Donnell MA. Use of intravesical BCG in treatment of superficial bladder cancer. In: Droller MJ, editor. Bladder cancer: current diagnosis and treatment. Totowa (NJ): Humana Press; 2001. p. 225–6.

[32] Witjes JA. Bladder carcinoma in situ in 2003: state of the art. Eur Urol 2004;45:142–6.

[33] Shelley MD, Wilt TJ, Court J, et al. Intravesical bacillus Calmette-Guerin is superior to mitomycin C in reducing tumour recurrence in high-risk superficial bladder cancer: a meta-analysis of randomized trials. BJU Int 2004;93:485–90.

[34] Bohle A, Jocham D, Bock PR. Intravesical bacillus Calmette-Guerin versus mitomycin C for superficial bladder cancer: a formal meta-analysis of comparative studies on recurrence and toxicity. J Urol 2003; 169:90–5.

[35] Huncharek M, Kupelnick B. Impact of intravesical chemotherapy versus BCG immunotherapy on recurrence of superficial transitional cell carcinoma of the bladder: meta-analytic re-evaluation. Am J Clin Oncol 2003;26:402–7.

[36] Sylvester RJ, van der Meijden AP, Lamm DL. Intravesical bacillus Calmette-Guerin reduces the risk of progression in patients with superficial bladder cancer: a meta-analysis of the published results of randomized clinical trials. J Urol 2002;168:1964–70.

[37] Bohle A, Bock PR. Intravesical bacille Calmette-Guerin versus mitomycin C in superficial bladder cancer: formal meta-analysis of comparative studies on tumor progression. Urology 2004;63:682–6.

[38] Luftenegger W, Ackermann DK, Futterlieb A, et al. Intravesical versus intravesical plus intradermal bacillus Calmette-Guerin: a prospective randomized study in patients with recurrent superficial bladder tumors. J Urol 1996;155:483–7.

[39] Kelley DR, Ratliff TL, Catalona WJ, et al. Intravesical bacillus Calmette-Guerin therapy for superficial bladder cancer: effect of bacillus Calmette-Guerin viability on treatment results. J Urol 1985;134: 48–53.

[40] Mack D, Frick J. Five-year results of a phase II study with low-dose bacille Calmette-Guerin therapy in high risk superficial bladder cancer. Urology 1995; 45:958–61.

[41] Hurle R, Losa A, Ranieri A, et al. Low dose Pasteur bacillus Calmette-Guerin regimen in stage T1, grade 3 bladder cancer therapy. J Urol 1996;156: 1602–5.

[42] Pagano F, Bassi P, Milani C, et al. A low dose bacillus Calmette-Guerin regimen in superficial bladder cancer therapy: is it effective? J Urol 1991;146:32–5.

[43] Martinez-Pineiro JA, Flores N, Isorna S, et al for CUETO (Club Urologico Espanol de Tratamiento Oncologico). Long-term follow-up of a randomized prospective trial comparing a standard 81 mg dose of intravesical bacille Calmette-Guerin with a reduced dose of 27 mg in superficial bladder cancer. BJU Int 2002;89:671–80.

[44] Morales A, Nickel JA, Wilson JW. Dose-response of bacillus Calmette-Guerin in the treatment of superficial bladder cancer. J Urol 1992;147:1256–8.

[45] Hudson MA, Ratliff TL, Gillen DP, et al. Single course versus maintenance bacillus Calmette-Guerin therapy for superficial bladder tumors: a prospective, randomized trial. J Urol 1987;138:295–8.

[46] Badalament RA, Herr HW, Wong GY, et al. A prospective randomized trial of maintenance versus nonmaintenance intravesical bacillus Calmette-Guerin therapy of superficial bladder cancer. J Clin Oncol 1987;5:441–9.

[47] Lamm DL, Blumenstein BA, Crissman JD, et al. Maintenance BCG immunotherapy in recurrent Ta, T1 and carcinoma in situ transitional cell carcinoma: a randomized Southwest Oncology Group study. J Urol 2000;163:1124–9.

[48] Saint F, Irani J, Patard JJ, et al. Tolerability of bacille Calmette-Guerin maintenance therapy for superficial bladder cancer. Urology 2001;57:883–8.

[49] Kolodziej A, Dembowski J, Zdrojowy R, et al. Treatment of high-risk superficial bladder cancer with maintenance bacille Calmette-Guerin therapy: preliminary results. BJU Int 2002;89:620–2.

[50] van der Meijden AP, Sylvester RJ, Oosterlinck W, et al. EORTC Genito-Urinary Tract Cancer Group. Maintenance bacillus Calmette-Guerin for Ta T1 bladder tumors is not associated with increased toxicity: results from a European Organisation for Research and Treatment of Cancer Genito-Urinary Group Phase III Trial. Eur Urol 2003;44:429–34.

[51] Bassi P, Spinadin R, Carando R, et al. Modified induction course: a solution to side effects? Eur Urol 2000;37(Suppl 1):31–2.

[52] Malmstrom PU, Wijkstrom H, Lundholm C, et al. 5-Year follow-up of a randomized prospective study comparing mitomycin C and bacillus Calmette-Guerin in patients with superficial bladder carcinoma: Swedish-Norwegian Bladder Cancer Study Group. J Urol 1999;161:1124–7.

[53] Brake M, Loertzer H, Horsch R, et al. Long-term results of intravesical bacillus Calmette-Guerin therapy for stage T1 superficial bladder cancer. Urology 2000;55:673–8.

[54] Pansadoro V, De Paula F. Intravesical bacillus Calmette-Guerin in the treatment of superficial transitional cell carcinoma of the bladder. J Urol 1987; 138:299–301.

[55] Heney NM, Ahmed S, Flanagan MJ, et al. Superficial bladder cancer: progression and recurrence. J Urol 1983;130:1083–6.

[56] Lutzeyer W, Rubben H, Dahm H. Prognostic parameters in superficial bladder cancer: an analysis of 315 cases. J Urol 1982;127:250–2.

[57] Catalona WJ, Hudson MA, Gillen DP, et al. Risks and benefits of repeated courses of intravesical bacillus Calmette-Guerin therapy for superficial bladder cancer. J Urol 1987;137:220–4.

[58] Belldegrun AS, Franklin JR, O'Donnell MA, et al. Superficial bladder cancer: the role of interferon-alpha. J Urol 1998;159:1793–801.

[59] Torti FM, Shortliffe LD, Williams RD, et al. Alpha-interferon in superficial bladder cancer: a Northern California Oncology Group Study. J Clin Oncol 1988;6:476–83.

[60] Giannakopoulos S, Gekas A, Alivizatos G, et al. Efficacy of escalating doses of intravesical interferon alpha-2b in reducing recurrence rate and progression in superficial transitional cell carcinoma. Br J Urol 1998;82:829–34.

[61] Malmstrom PU. A randomized comparative dose-ranging study of interferon-alpha and mitomycin-C as an internal control in primary or recurrent superficial transitional cell carcinoma. BJU Int 2001; 89:681–6.

[62] Portillo J, Martin B, Hernandez R, et al. Results at 43 months' follow-up of a double-blind, randomized, prospective clinical trial using intravesical interferon alpha-2b in the prophylaxis of stage pT1 transitional cell carcinoma of the bladder. Urology 1997;49:187–90.

[63] Jimenez-Cruz JF, Vera-Donoso CD, Leiva O, et al. Intravesical immunoprophylaxis in recurrent superficial bladder cancer (stage T1): multicenter trial comparing bacille Calmette-Guerin and interferon-alpha. Urology 1997;50:529–35.

[64] Williams RD, Gleason DM, Smith AY, et al. Pilot study of intravesical alfa-2b interferon for treatment of bladder carcinoma in situ following BCG failure. J Urol 1996;155:494A.

[65] Lam JS, Benson MC, O'Donnell MA, et al. Bacillus Calmette-Guerin plus interferon-alpha2B intravesical therapy maintains an extended treatment plan for superficial bladder cancer with minimal toxicity. Urol Oncol 2003;21:354–60.

[66] Punnen SP, Chin JL, Jewett MAS. Management of bacillus Calmette-Guerin (BCG) refractory superficial bladder cancer: results with intravesical BCG and interferon combination therapy. Can J Urol 2003;10:1790–5.

[67] O'Donnell MA, Krohn J, DeWolf WC. Salvage intravesical therapy with interferon-α-2B plus low dose bacillus Calmette-Guerin is effective in patients with superficial bladder cancer in whom bacillus Calmette-Guerin alone previously failed. J Urol 2001;166:1300–5.

[68] O'Donnell MA, Lilli K, Leopold C. National Bacillus Calmette-Guerin/Interferon Phase 2 Investigator Group: interim results from a national multicenter phase II trial of combination bacillus Calmette-Guerin plus interferon alfa-2b for superficial bladder cancer. J Urol 2004;172:888–93.

[69] Steinberg G, Bahnson R, Brosman S, et al. Efficacy and safety of valrubicin for the treatment of bacillus Calmette-Guerin refractory carcinoma in situ of the bladder: the Valrubicin Study Group. J Urol 2000; 163:761–7.

[70] Calabro F, Sternberg CN. New drugs and new approaches for the treatment of metastatic urothelial cancer. World J Urol 2002;20:158–66.

[71] Le Visage C, Rioux-Leclercq N, Haller M, et al. Efficacy of paclitaxel released from bio-adhesive polymer microspheres on model superficial bladder cancer. J Urol 2004;171:1324–9.

[72] Laufer M, Ramalingam S, Schoenberg MP, et al. Intravesical gemcitabine therapy for superficial transitional cell carcinoma of the bladder: a phase I and pharmacokinetic study. J Clin Oncol 2003;21: 697–703.

[73] Dalbagni G, Russo P, Sheinfeld J, et al. Phase I trial of intravesical gemcitabine in bacillus Calmette-Guerin-refractory transitional-cell carcinoma of the bladder. J Clin Oncol 2002;20:3193–8.

[74] De Berardinis E, Antonini G, Peters GJ, et al. Intravesical administration of gemcitabine in superficial bladder cancer: a phase I study with pharmacodynamic evaluation. BJU Int 2004;93:491–4.

[75] Gontero P, Casetta G, Maso G, et al. Phase II study to investigate the ablative efficacy of intravesical administration of gemcitabine in intermediate-risk superficial bladder cancer (SBC). Eur Urol 2004; 46:339–43.

[76] Dalbagni G, Mazumdar M, Russo P, et al. Phase II trial of intravesical gemcitabine in BCG-refractory transitional cell carcinoma of the bladder. J Urol 2004;171:274A.

[77] Maymi J, Saltsgaver N, O'Donnell MA. New intravesical sequential chemotherapy for patients with treatment refractory superficial urothelial carcinoma. Poster presentation at meeting of Proc Soc Urol Oncol 2004.

[78] Colombo R, Da Pozzo LF, Salonia A, et al. Multicentric study comparing intravesical chemotherapy alone and with local microwave hyperthermia for prophylaxis of recurrence of superficial transitional cell carcinoma. J Clin Oncol 2003;21:4270–6.

[79] Colombo R, Da Pozzo LF, Lev A, et al. Local microwave hyperthermia and intravesical chemotherapy as bladder sparing treatment for select multifocal and unresectable superficial bladder tumors. J Urol 1998;159:783–7.

[80] Gofrit ON, Shapiro A, Pode D, et al. Combined local bladder hyperthermia and intravesical chemotherapy for the treatment of high-grade superficial bladder cancer. Urology 2004;63:466–71.

[81] van der Heijden AG, Kiemeney LA, Gofrit ON, et al. Preliminary European results of local microwave hyperthermia and chemotherapy treatment in intermediate or high risk superficial transitional cell carcinoma of the bladder. Eur Urol 2004;46:65–71.

[82] Di Stasi SM, Giannantoni A, Stephen RL, et al. Intravesical electromotive mitomycin C versus passive transport mitomycin C for high risk superficial bladder cancer: a prospective randomized study. J Urol 2003;170:777–82.

[83] Waidelich R, Stepp H, Baumgartner R, et al. Clinical experience with 5-aminolevulinic acid and photodynamic therapy for refractory superficial bladder cancer. J Urol 2001;165:1904–7.

[84] Berger AP, Steiner H, Stenzl A, et al. Photodynamic therapy with intravesical instillation of 5-aminolevulinic acid for patients with recurrent superficial bladder cancer: a single-center study. Urology 2003;61: 338–41.

[85] Kamuhabwa A, Agostinis P, Ahmed B, et al. Hypericin as a potential phototherapeutic agent in superficial transitional cell carcinoma of the bladder. Photochem Photobiol Sci 2004;3:772–80.

ELSEVIER
SAUNDERS

Urol Clin N Am 32 (2005) 133–145

UROLOGIC
CLINICS
of North America

Optimal Management of the T1G3 Bladder Cancer

Murugesan Manoharan, MD, FRCS(Eng), FRACS(Urol), Mark S. Soloway, MD*

Department of Urology, University of Miami School of Medicine, 1400 NW 10th Avenue, # 506, Miami, FL 33136, USA

Management decisions for a patient with a high-grade T1 urothelial cancer of the bladder are both critical and controversial. In the authors' view, if one uses a grading scale of 0 to 10 for difficulty in decision making (10 being the most difficult), the patient with T1G3 tumor rates a 10.

By definition, these high-grade bladder tumors invade the lamina propria without involving the muscularis propria [1]. They have high propensity for recurrence and progression. Following trans-urethral resection (TURBT) of the initial T1G3 tumor with no additional therapy, there is a recurrence rate of 50% to 70% and a progression rate of 25% to 50% [2,3].

The optimal management of these tumors requires an accurate diagnosis including the stage and grade, and careful assessment of prognostic factors. The wide range of available treatment options includes TURBT alone, adding intravesical therapy, radical cystectomy, and even possibly chemoradiation. Despite advances in the understanding of the biologic behavior of these tumors, both the choice and timing of treatment remain controversial [3].

Diagnosis, evaluation, and initial management

The initial critical step is to establish an accurate diagnosis. An inaccurate diagnosis, particularly understaging, can adversely impact the survival of the patient. Overtreatment affects the quality of life and possibly leads to unnecessary morbidity. This is precisely why the decision making is so difficult.

---

* Corresponding author.
  E-mail address: msoloway@miami.edu
(M.S. Soloway).

Thorough endoscopic evaluation of the bladder followed by complete excision of all visible tumors should be performed. To avoid staging errors, cautery artifact should be minimized. It is imperative to have muscle from the muscularis propria in the specimen and some advocate cold cup biopsies of the tumor base [4]. Tumor resection is improved by using a videoendoscope with continuous flow. Some advocate the use of fluorescence endoscopy using 5-alpha aminolevulinic acid to facilitate complete resection and identification of carcinoma in situ [5]. The authors have not used this.

Herr [6] retrospectively evaluated the concordance of the pathologic diagnoses between an initial resection and a second TURBT in 150 patients. The results of the second resection changed the treatment in 33% of these patients. He emphasized the importance of obtaining muscle in the resected specimen. Of 23 patients with a T1 lesion without muscle in the first resection, 11 (49%) were upstaged to T2 after obtaining information from the second TURBT. A caveat of this study is that not only did different urologists perform the first and second TURBTs, but different pathologists read the first and second bladder tumor specimens. Dutta et al [7] similarly reported a 64% risk of understaging T1 lesions when muscle was absent compared with only 30% when muscle was present in the TURBT specimen.

Can the urologist be confident that the TURBT removed the entire tumor? Clearly the experience of the urologist is critical but there are many variables. Zurkirchen et al [8] retrospectively reviewed those patients who underwent follow-up TURBTs within 6 weeks of the initial resection. A total of 37% had persistent tumor on the second resection. Grimm et al [9] similarly retrospectively reviewed 83 patients who underwent a repeat TURBT a mean of 7 weeks after the initial TURBT. Residual tumor was found in 33%. On univariate analysis, tumor stage and grade were identified as predictive for residual tumor on restaging TURBT. Furthermore, there was a significant decrease in 5-year disease-free survival between those who underwent a second TURBT and those who did not (63% and 40%, respectively). Both multifocality and tumor grade increased the risk of finding residual tumor on a second TURBT. There are no studies available at present regarding the optimal timing of the second resection. The consensus is, however, that this should be performed within 1 to 4 weeks following the initial resection. May et al [10] and Sanchez-Oritz et al [11] reported that a delay of more than 12 weeks in muscle-invasive bladder cancer leads to significant upstaging. Undue delay in second resection should be avoided.

Abnormal-looking urothelium should be biopsied. The role of random bladder biopsy is controversial, however, and there is no strong evidence currently to support this [12–15]. Whenever cold cup biopsies are performed it is advisable to fulgurate the biopsy sites to prevent bleeding [16]. Bladder wash cytology is an integral part of the second endoscopic session because it provides a representative mini biopsy from the entire bladder urothelium and may be particularly helpful if there is no visible tumor yet there are cancer cells in the cytology.

These studies show that the risk of upstaging on second TURBT is at least 30% if muscle is present in the specimen and even higher if muscle is not present. Further, the risk of residual tumor on second TURBT is also significant. Even for solitary, papillary-appearing tumors, the risk is 24% to 27% and it is higher for multifocal, nonpapillary lesions. The authors recommend that a second TURBT be considered in patients with a T1G3 tumor. The authors do not always perform a second resection. Most patients who present to the authors with a high-grade T1 tumor have had the initial resection elsewhere and a second resection (the authors' first) is performed. If the authors perform a first resection and the tumor is small, has a minimal lamina propria invasion, and muscle is clearly present and uninvolved, they do not perform a second TUR. Nonetheless, most of the time, they perform a second TURBT.

Attempts have been made further to substage T1 tumors. Holmang et al [17] retrospectively reviewed 121 patients with T1G3 bladder cancers and evaluated whether the tumors invaded above the level of the muscularis mucosae (stage T1a) or invaded into and beyond it (stage T1b). A total of 54% of patients were categorized as T1a and 40% as T1b; only 6% of patients could not be substaged. Stage T1b tumors were more likely to progress following the initial TUR; 58% of those with grade 3 T1b tumors progressed to muscle-invasive disease compared with only 36% with grade 3 T1a tumors. The 5-year overall survival for T1a and T1b tumors was 54% and 42%, respectively. Hasui et al [18] similarly reported a worse prognosis if the T1 tumor invaded the muscularis mucosae. With a mean follow-up of 78 months, the progression rates for T1a and T1b cancers were 7% and 54%, respectively. Moreover, the increase risk of progression was seen regardless of the grade, size, or multifocality of the tumor. Smits et al [19] categorized T1 tumors into T1a, T1b, and T1c (up to, into, and beyond the muscularis mucosae, respectively) and retrospectively evaluated the risk of recurrence and progression among the three groups. There was no difference in the 3-year risk of recurrence between the three groups; however, the risk of progression was 6%, 33%, and 55%, respectively. Furthermore, if the pathology was T1c and associated carcinoma in situ the risk of progression was 27 times compared with those without T1c and carcinoma in situ. Despite these reports, this substaging system has not been widely adopted because muscularis mucosae are often absent or difficult to identify. The authors' pathologists usually provide this information.

Cheng et al [20] measured the depth of invasion to substage T1 tumors, to obviate the difficulty in identifying the muscularis mucosae. They retrospectively reviewed 55 patients with T1 bladder cancer. TURBT specimens were evaluated for depth of stromal invasion, as measured with a micrometer from the basement membrane to the deepest tumor cells. There was a significant correlation between the depth of invasion in the TURBT specimen and the stage at cystectomy. Using a cutoff of greater than 1.5 mm depth of invasion, the sensitivity, specificity, and positive and negative predictive values for predicting advanced stage disease ($>$T2) were 81%, 83%, 95%, and 56%, respectively.

Prognostic factors

Various prognostic factors associated with T1G3 tumors should be carefully identified and evaluated. These greatly assist the physician in the decision-making process. The most accepted predictors of progression in patients with T1G3 bladder tumors are clinical and pathologic. The response to intravesical therapy is a reliable predictor of progression that can be assessed at 3 to 9 months [21–23]. After analyzing the outcome in 191 patients with stage T1 disease with or without carcinoma in situ, Solsona et al [23] reported that 80% who were not free of cancer at 3 months had progression. They also indicated that high grade, association of carcinoma in situ, and prostate mucosa or duct involvement represent significant pathologic predictors of progression. Tumor size, multiplicity, and vascular invasion are other important prognostic factors [24].

A variety of biologic markers have been studied as a prognostic marker for T1 disease. It seems that T1G3 tumors behave as bacillus Calmette-Guérin (BCG) sensitive, responding to treatment after initial therapy, or BCG refractory, continuing to recur or progress despite BCG. Efforts have been made to define predictors for the response to BCG or patients at high risk for progression. The p53 tumor suppresser gene is a commonly altered gene in human malignancies. In a series of 60 patients with bladder cancer Pfister et al [25] observed mutant p53 in 66% of stage T1 grade 3 but in no stage Ta grade 1 tumor. Tumors with mutant p53 inactivate transcription of p21 and the Bax gene. Alterations of p53 were associated with BCG failure. Others have not found that p53 expression correlates with BCG failure [26–28]. Controversial results have also been reported in regard to p53 expression as an independent predictor of progression. In a case-control study Llopis et al [29] showed that p53 expression analyzed at a cutoff of 20% positivity is a significant predictor of progression. Others have also reported this finding [30,31]. Steiner et al [32] did not note that p53 status was helpful for selecting candidates for radical cystectomy. Lopez-Beltran et al [33] reported a number of cell cycle regulators, such as p27kip1, cyclin D1, and cyclin D3, which are independent predictors. None of these factors can accurately predict the biologic behavior of a T1G3 tumor and hence the search for more reliable prognostic indicators continues.

Intravesical therapy

Following TUR of a high-grade T1 tumor, the risk of recurrence approaches 80% and the risk of progression is 50% to 65% [2,3]. The goals of adjuvant intravesical therapy are to decrease the rate of recurrence and ultimately decrease the chance of progression. Although low-grade tumors recur frequently but rarely progress, high-grade tumors or tumors that invade the lamina propria are potentially lethal. Intravesical therapy with chemotherapeutic or immunologic agents in an adjuvant fashion after endoscopic resection has been shown to decrease the recurrence rate of stages Ta and T1 transitional cell carcinoma of the bladder.

Immunotherapy

BCG is believed by many groups to be the most effective agent for treating carcinoma in situ and high-grade stage Ta or T1 transitional cell carcinoma [34–36]. To the authors' knowledge, the precise mechanism remains unclear. It seems that BCG must be in contact with tumor cells through novel receptors [37]. This contact results in a local immunologic host response, generating a T-helper cell response and immunocompetent cytotoxic T-cell activation. Data also suggest that during this process cytokines, such as interleukins, are released and exert antineoplastic activity [38–41]. In contemporary series of T1G3 tumors, the recurrence rate after TUR and intravesical BCG is 23% to 74% [41–43]. After analyzing the outcome of a series of 51 patients with stage T1G3 tumors treated with adjuvant BCG, Hurle et al [44] reported a recurrence rate of 25% at a median follow-up of 85 months. A higher recurrence rate of 44% was reported by Cookson and Sarosdy [41], who followed 86 patients with T1 tumors (mean = 59 months). In a series of 44 patients with T1G3 tumors and a mean follow-up of 28 months Brake et al [42] reported a 27% recurrence rate after TUR and adjuvant BCG. Controlled studies comparing TUR alone versus TUR and BCG indicate an almost 40% decrease in tumor recurrence with adjuvant therapy [41,44]. Most controlled studies enrolled patients with both Ta and T1 tumors [45–49]. In an analysis of more than 30 randomized controlled trials, the American Urological Association Bladder Cancer Clinical Guidelines Panel noted that intravesical BCG after TUR decreases the recurrence rate by 30% compared with TUR alone [50]. Furthermore, the guidelines panel stated that BCG and mitomycin C are superior to doxorubicin and thiotepa. In a randomized prospective study comparing mitomycin C with BCG, Malmström et al [35] noted that BCG was superior to mitomycin C for prophylaxis. This finding was more evident in the group of patients with nonpapillary tumors or carcinoma in situ. No difference was observed in progression or survival. This study validated the previous results of Lundholm et al [51], who reported significantly longer time to treatment failure for BCG than for mitomycin C. To the authors' knowledge, the optimal dose and schedule of intravesical BCG have not been established. The most commonly used regimen of 6 weekly doses is arbitrary. The induction phase required for an efficient immune response may occur with fewer doses, although some patients may require more than 6 weekly doses. There is a suggestion that a lower dose of BCG is not as effective for high-grade cancer [52,53].

Maintenance bacillus Calmette-Guérin therapy

The Southwest Oncology Group reported promising results in a combined series of patients with stages Ta and T1 bladder tumors at high risk, using a maintenance protocol consisting of a 6-week induction course of BCG followed by three weekly instillations at 3 and 6 months, and every 6 months thereafter for 3 years. The limited number of patients (16%) who tolerated the maintenance BCG therapy to complete the 3-year program represents a significant drawback of this regimen [54,55]. This regimen seems promising, however, and at the present time most urologists believe that some maintenance BCG therapy is advisable.

Intravesical chemotherapy

Mitomycin C seems to be the most effective initial adjuvant intravesical chemotherapeutic agent for stages Ta and T1 bladder cancer [41,56]. Mitomycin C is an alkylating agent that binds to DNA, resulting in synthesis inhibition and strand breakage [57,58]. To the authors' knowledge there is no standard regimen for instilling mitomycin C and there has never been a proper dose-response study. When used to treat residual tumor, the drug is usually administered weekly for 6 to 8 weeks. The dose is 20 to 40 mg [59]. Substantial evidence suggests that tumor cell implantation is a cause of early tumor recurrence and may be influenced by a single dose of mitomycin C within 24 hours after TUR [60,61]. Other intravesical chemotherapeutic agents that have been shown to be beneficial for the prophylaxis of recurrence are thiotepa, doxorubicin, and epirubicin. Although intravesical treatment

has been beneficial for decreasing the recurrence rate, this treatment has not decreased the chance of progression [57,58]. Others have suggested combining two chemotherapeutic agents. Isaka et al [61] treated 40 patients with stage T2 or less bladder cancer with a combination of mitomycin and doxorubicin. They achieved a 45% complete response in 20 patients treated for multiple recurrences. The tumor-free recurrence rate in 20 patients treated for prophylaxis after TUR was 66% at a mean follow-up of 14 months. Using the same intravesical combination in two regimens (with and without 1 year of maintenance) Fukui et al [62] observed that the maintenance regimen was beneficial for carcinoma in situ only. Despite a slightly better outcome, especially in patients with carcinoma in situ, combination chemotherapy resulted in a modest outcome improvement with increased local side effects.

Randomized, prospective trials demonstrate that the risk of recurrence can be reduced by 50% at 2 years and at least by 15% at 5 years with a single dose of immediate instillation of mitomycin following TUR [63–65]. It is also recommended that the single-dose mitomycin should be given within 6 hours but no more than 24 hours following TUR. If mitomycin is given within 24 hours following TUR, maintenance intravesical chemotherapy does not significantly reduce the recurrence further [66].

Following a TUR for a T1G3 tumor the authors recommend instilling a single dose of mitomycin within 24 hours. They instill this in the recovery room following the TUR. The catheter is clamped for 1 hour. This cannot be done if there is bleeding or perforation. This should be followed by a standard 6-week course of BCG. Maintenance BCG therapy (Southwest Oncology Group regimen) seems to be useful. Three months following the TUR and intravesical therapy, the authors perform a flexible cystoscopy and bladder wash cytology. Presence of tumor or positive cytology requires further careful evaluation including resection of the tumor, biopsies of the bladder mucosa, and prostatic urethra depending on the findings.

Treatment options after bacillus Calmette-Guérin failure

Although BCG is an effective adjuvant treatment for T1G3 bladder cancer, approximately 50% of patients recur and 15% to 50% of patients progress within the first 5 years following BCG therapy (Table 1) [67–74]. Interpreting the results from many of the studies is difficult because of differences in the definition of BCG failure.

Herr and Dalbagni [75] define the "BCG refractory state" as the failure to achieve a disease-free state by 6 months after initial BCG therapy with either maintenance or retreatment at 3 months because of either persistence or recurrent disease. "BCG relapse" refers to recurrence after achieving disease-free status at 6 months. The "BCG intolerance" refers to discontinuation of the therapy because of side effects and should be considered as true BCG failures.

Radical cystectomy is the most appropriate option for patients who recur with high-grade or high-stage disease. A patient's personal preference and comorbidity, however, may require an alternative treatment strategy. The treatment for BCG failure starts with a complete repeat resection of all visible tumors. The options following resection include the following.

Repeat bacillus Calmette-Guérin therapy

There are insufficient data in the literature on the effectiveness of repeat BCG therapy. Cookson and Sarosdy [41] reported excellent results with a response rate of 64% in patients with T1 recurrence following TUR and repeat BCG. Brake et al [69] reported a 51% response rate in BCG-refractory patients, but 30% of patients in this group progressed to muscle-invasive disease. Pansadoro et al [76] report an inferior response rate of 27% following TUR and a second 6-week course of BCG and even poorer response rate of 6% following a third cycle of BCG. The authors reserve repeat BCG therapy for selected patients who recur with low-grade or low-stage transitional cell

carcinoma and these patients need aggressive surveillance.

Intravesical chemotherapy

Although intravesical treatment with chemotherapeutic agents, such as mitomycin C, is an option, there are little data regarding its role in recurrent T1G3 tumors following BCG failure. Response rates of 19% and 21% with mitomycin and valrubicin are among the few reports [77,78]. These results are poor and the authors do not recommend intravesical salvage chemotherapy especially for patients with T1G3 following BCG.

Interferon therapy

The long-term efficacy with interferon-α monotherapy is less than 15% [79] and hence this therapy is unlikely to benefit BCG failure patients particularly with a T1G3 cancer. There are several reports, however, which confirm the substantial synergistic benefit of BCG plus interferon combination therapy in BCG failure cases. The disease-free rates range from 50% to 60% and more importantly no one had unresectable or metastatic disease at cystectomy following BCG-interferon combination therapy [80,81]. In a multi-institutional study, O'Donnell et al [82] showed a response rate of 42% at a median follow-up of 24 months. The authors have used this combination for some patients who have recurred after BCG and it is well tolerated.

Radiation therapy and photodynamic therapy

The role of radiation as a salvage option for BCG failure is unknown. The reported 5-year disease-free survival rate is 50%, however, in patients with high-grade T1 urothelial cancer

Table 1
Results of TUR plus BCG for T1G3 tumors

Series/year	No. patients	Follow-up (mo)	Recurrence (%)	Progression (%)
Pfister (1995)	26	54	50	27
Lebret (1998)	35	45	43	20
Brake (2000)	44	43	27	16
Patard (2001)	50	65	52	22
Kulkarni (2002)	69	48	46	12
Bogdanovic (2002)	43	53	28	16
Peyromaure (2003)	57	53	42	23
Shanin (2003)	92	64	70	33

Abbreviations: BCG, bacille Calmette-Guérin; TUR, transurethral resection.

treated with external beam radiation [83]. More-over, for T1 disease, the local recurrence and progression rates are approximately 50% [84]. These results are inferior to radical cystectomy and the authors do not recommend radiation ther-apy if the subsequent tumor is high-grade Ta or T1. Photodynamic therapy with 5-aminolevulinic acid may have a role in carcinoma in situ but there are no studies confirming its benefit in BCG failure with T1 disease [85].

Role of cystectomy: early versus deferred

The timing of cystectomy is a most debated issue in the management of T1G3 tumors. Despite intravesical adjuvant therapies, there is a substan-tial group of patients with initial high-grade stage T1 tumor who have progression and are at risk of dying from urothelial cancer [86].

Several groups recommend immediate or early cystectomy without a trial of adjuvant intravesical therapy with or without repeat TUR. Supporters of this approach argue that the 5-year survival rate of 90% may decrease to 50% to 60% if radical cystectomy is delayed until progression [87]. Apart from this, there are several valid arguments that support both early and deferred cystectomy.

Conservative management with TUR and intravesical treatment is associated with continu-ous decline in survival with lifelong risk of re-currence, progression, and metastasis [88]. Shahin et al [74] reported that in a series of 153 patients, following TUR and BCG for a T1G3 tumor the recurrence rate was 75% after 10 years. Further-more, their analysis indicated a continuous decline in survival with an estimated 30% of patients dead at 10 years. Herr [89], in is his editorial, stressed the fact that this is a high figure for a newly diagnosed non–muscle invasive bladder cancer. Currently, there are not reliable markers that can differentiate patients who recur from those who do not. On the basis of modern molecular techniques including comparative ge-nomic hybridization, fluorescence in situ hybrid-ization, and microarray expression, both T1 and T2 disease share the same gene alteration (chro-mosome 17) that specifies the invasive ability of the tumor [90].

The initial diagnosis of T1 disease is associated with significant understaging errors of as much as 25% to 40%. Delay in offering the correct treatment, such as cystectomy, affects the survival. In a series of 189 patients who underwent

cystectomy within 3 months of diagnosis of muscle-invasive disease, there was a significantly better 5-year progression-free survival than if cystectomy was performed more than 3 months following diagnosis (55% and 34%, respectively) [10].

Herr and Sogani [91] retrospectively evaluated 90 patients with high-risk superficial bladder cancer who ultimately underwent cystectomy. They demonstrated improved 15-year disease-specific survival for those who underwent cystec-tomy within 2 years after initial BCG treatment. Those who underwent cystectomy for recurrent superficial disease had better outcome than those who underwent surgery for progression. They concluded that deferring cystectomy until pro-gression to muscle-invasive disease may decrease the overall disease-specific survival. A total of 217 patients from their original cohort of 307 with high-risk superficial disease never required cystec-tomy, however, and were spared the morbidity of cystectomy.

Conservative management has a disadvantage of rigorous lifelong follow-up with cystoscopy and imaging studies apart from need for further adjuvant therapy for recurrences. The social im-plications and financial burden on the health system should be considered. Advancement in urinary diversion techniques has improved the quality of life. Hart et al [92] studied the quality of life following cystectomy and reported excellent overall quality of life; minimal emotional distress; and no significant problems with social, physical, and functional activities. Recently, Henningsohn et al [93] studied the quality of life in a series of 101 patients (patients who are recurrence free after cystectomy and orthotopic neobladder sub-stitution) and compared it with a matched control group. This study highlighted that the quality of life issues including sexual function and urinary leakage were similar. As a whole, the contempo-rary cystectomy in both genders has adapted several techniques to preserve quality of life [88].

Because the progression rate is approximately 25% with TUR plus BCG and 50% with TUR alone, it seems that with early cystectomy at least 50% of patients are overtreated. Furthermore, the morbidity and mortality associated with radical cystectomy are 20% and 1% to 4%, respectively [94]. Despite techniques of orthotopic bladder replacement the quality of life is altered to a certain extent. It is reasonable, however, to offer immediate cystectomy to young patients with deep T1 tumors (>1.5 mm in depth) with at least one additional bad prognostic factor (Box 1) including multifocality, carcinoma in situ, involvement of the prostate, and anatomic difficulties in TUR [88].

The most important issue is how to restrict radical cystectomy to selective patients at high risk and to choose an initial bladder-sparing approach in others without affecting survival. In most cases this goal can be achieved by combining complete TUR with BCG adjuvant therapy, while being prepared to recognize the appropriate time for radical cystectomy.

Recent advances in treatment options

Several studies are underway at various stages that are likely to impact in future the treatment options available to treat T1G3 tumor.

Sequential Intravesical therapy

To improve the efficacy of the intravesical therapy, several alternative approaches combining BCG with chemotherapeutic agents are being investigated. The rationale for giving immediate post–tumor resection chemotherapy before BCG is to reduce tumor implantation and to induce sloughing of the urothelium, allowing BCG to interact better with fibronectin and initiating an immune response. Soloway et al [95] suggested that complete resection of the tumor followed by immediate mitomycin C instillation and six weekly BGG instillations results in an acceptably low recurrence and progression rate.

Sequential regimen using drugs with different mechanism of action may be beneficial because of synergistic effect and may be well tolerated. In a randomized study of 188 patients with rapidly recurrent stages Ta and T1 transitional cell carcinoma, Rintala et al [96] compared mitomycin C alone with mitomycin C and BCG. At a mean follow-up of 34 months no difference was observed in terms of tumor recurrence and disease-

free interval. A similar comparison was performed in the randomized phase III protocol of Witjes et al [97]. In this study patients were randomized to 10 instillations of mitomycin C or 4 instillations of mitomycin C followed by 6 weeks of BCG. No significant difference was observed in the two regimens in regard to recurrence, progression, or systemic toxicity. Randomized prospective studies show that sequential BCG and epirubicin is not more effective than BCG alone [98–100]. Serretta et al [101] reported using adjuvant sequential mitomycin C and epirubicin in 91 of 137 patients with T1G3 bladder cancer after initial TUR. With close to 20 years of follow-up overall recurrence rate was less in the sequential chemotherapy protocol but the overall progression rate was similar (9.5%). The cystectomy rate was 7% and the disease-specific death rate was 7%. Despite various studies it is still not proved that the sequential chemotherapy is superior to BCG monotherapy.

Newer intravesical agents

Gemcitabine and paclitaxel are promising intravesical chemotherapeutic agents currently at different stages of investigation. In a phase I study, Dalbagni et al [102] reported that intravesical gemcitabine was well tolerated with minimal bladder irritation and acceptable myelosuppression. Serum levels of gemcitabine were undetectable at concentrations of 5, 10, and 15 mg/mL. Serum gemcitabine was detected, however, at a concentration of 20 mg/mL. A complete response (negative posttreatment cystoscopy including a biopsy of the urothelium and a negative cytology) was achieved in 7 (39%) of 18 patients. In a phase II study of patients with BCG-refractory transitional cell carcinoma to determine the efficacy of gemcitabine as an intravesical agent, 28 patients completed therapy, and 16 achieved a complete response [103]. All the recent studies confirm that gemcitabine is an effective intravesical agent, with low systemic absorption and little systemic and local toxicity [104,105].

Paclitaxel is in the early stages of testing. In vitro studies showed that a 2-hour exposure to cancer cells has significant anticancer potency [106]. The intravesical delivery is difficult, however, because of its lipid-soluble properties. Chemical modification of this drug may negate this property and allow better intravesical delivery [107].

Various other new strategies include gene therapy [108]; immunostimulants, such as mycobacterium cell wall DNA extract prepared from the *Mycobacterium phlei* [109]; growth factor–related signaling pathway modifiers [110]; and intravesical delivery of activated tumoricidal macrophages [111]. Recent advances in the intravesical delivery system for chemotherapeutic drugs include electromotive intravesical mitomycin C and mitomycin C in conjunction with local microwave hyperthermia. Both these methods show better tissue concentration and a statistically superior reduction in recurrence. Further studies are awaited [112,113].

Summary

T1G3 transitional cell carcinoma of the bladder represents a highly malignant tumor with a variable and unpredictable biologic potential. The most critical aspect of management requires a detailed discussion with the patient regarding the treatment options. Both the physician and the patient should be willing to reconsider the treatment options as the disease continues to evolve.

In most cases initial management involves complete resection of the tumor, accurate staging of the disease, and intravesical immunotherapy or chemotherapy. Rigorous surveillance with long-term follow-up is crucial for managing these cases. In selected cases with adverse prognostic factors immediate cystectomy should be considered. The choice and timing of the decision to abandon bladder preservation and proceed with cystectomy should be continuously reconsidered on an individual patient basis, in concordance with the evolution of the disease (Fig. 1). The goal is to spare the bladder when possible but not at the risk of death from metastatic disease. Radical cystectomy in high-grade stage T1 transitional cell carcinoma offers excellent results in regard to the prevention of recurrence and progression and survival. Improvements in urinary diversion and nerve-sparing techniques have decreased the magnitude of social implications related to cystectomy in most patients regardless of gender. The discovery of reliable

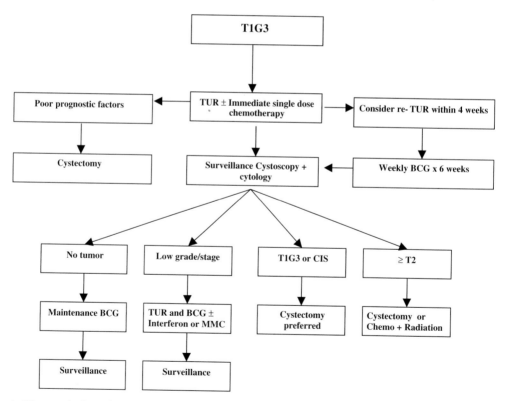

Fig. 1. Therapeutic flow chart for T1G3 tumors. BCG, bacille Calmette-Guérin; CIS, carcinoma in situ; MMC, mitomycin C; TUR, transurethral resection.

markers may contribute to better selection of patients for bladder sparing. Until then, the optimal treatment for the T1G3 tumor remains controversial.

References

[1] Patard J, Moudouni S, Saint F, et al. Tumor progression and survival in patients with T1G3 bladder tumors: multicentric retrospective study comparing 94 patients treated during 17 years. Urology 2001; 58:551–6.

[2] Jakse G, Loidl W, Seeber G, et al. Stage T1, grade 3 transitional cell carcinoma of the bladder: an unfavorable tumor? J Urol 1987;137:39–43.

[3] Amling CL, Thrasher JB, Frazier HA, et al. Radical cystectomy for stages Ta, Tis and T1 transitional cell carcinoma of the bladder. J Urol 1994; 151:31–5.

[4] Klan R, Loy V, Huland H. Residual tumor discovered in routine second transurethral resection in patients with stage T1 transitional cell carcinoma of the bladder. J Urol 1991;146:316–8.

[5] Zaak D, Hungerhuber E, Schneede P, et al. Role of 5-aminolevulinic acid in the detection of urothelial premalignant lesions. Cancer 2002;95:1234–8.

[6] Herr HW. The value of a second transurethral resection in evaluating patients with bladder tumors. J Urol 1999;162:74–6.

[7] Dutta SC, Smith JA Jr, Shappell SB, et al. Clinical under staging of high risk nonmuscle invasive urothelial carcinoma treated with radical cystectomy. J Urol 2001;166:490–3.

[8] Zurkirchen MA, Sulser T, Gaspert A, et al. Second transurethral resection of superficial transitional cell carcinoma of the bladder: a must even for experienced urologists. Urol Int 2004;72:99–102.

[9] Grimm MO, Steinhoff C, Simon X, et al. Effect of routine repeat transurethral resection for superficial bladder cancer: a long-term observational study. J Urol 2003;170(2 Pt 1):433–7.

[10] May M, Nitzke T, Helke C, et al. Significance of the time period between diagnosis of muscle invasion and radical cystectomy with regard to the prognosis of transitional cell carcinoma of the urothelium in the bladder. Scand J Urol Nephrol 2004;38:231–5.

[11] Sanchez-Ortiz RF, Huang WC, Mick R, et al. An interval longer than 12 weeks between the diagnosis of muscle invasion and cystectomy is associated with worse outcome in bladder carcinoma. J Urol 2003;169:110–5.

[12] Van Gils-Gielen RJ, Witjes WP, Caris CT, et al. Risk factors in carcinoma in situ of the urinary bladder. Dutch South East Cooperative Urological Group. Urology 1995;45:581–6.

[13] May F, Treiber U, Hartung R, et al. Significance of random bladder biopsies in superficial bladder cancer. Eur Urol 2003;44:47–50.

[14] Van der Meijden A, Oosterlinck W, Brausi M, et al. Significance of bladder biopsies in Ta, T1 bladder tumors: a report from the EORTC Genito-Urinary Tract Cancer Cooperative Group. EORTC-GU Group Superficial Bladder Committee. Eur Urol 1999;35:267–71.

[15] Taguchi I, Gohji K, Hara I, et al. Clinical evaluation of random biopsy of urinary bladder in patients with superficial bladder cancer. Int J Urol 1998;5:30–4.

[16] Levi AW, Potter SR, Schoenberg MP, et al. Clinical significance of denuded urothelium in bladder biopsy. J Urol 2001;166:457–60.

[17] Holmang S, Hedelin H, Anderstrom C, et al. The importance of the depth of invasion in stage T1 bladder carcinoma: a prospective cohort study. J Urol 1997;157:800–3.

[18] Hasui Y, Osada Y, Kitada S, et al. Significance of invasion to the muscularis mucosae on the progression of superficial bladder cancer. Urology 1994;43: 782–6.

[19] Smits G, Schaafsma E, Kiemeney L, et al. Microstaging of pT1 transitional cell carcinoma of the bladder: identification of subgroups with distinct risks of progression. Urology 1998;52:1009–13.

[20] Cheng L, Weaver AL, Neumann RM, et al. Substaging of T1 bladder carcinoma based on the depth of invasion as measured by micrometer: a new proposal. Cancer 1999;86:1035–43.

[21] Herr HW, Badalament RA, Amato DA, et al. Superficial bladder cancer treated with bacillus Calmette-Guérin: a multivariate analysis of factors affecting tumor progression. J Urol 1989;141:22.

[22] Merz VW, Marth D, Kraft R, et al. Analysis of early failures after intravesical instillation therapy with bacillus Calmette-Guérin for carcinoma in situ of the bladder. Br J Urol 1995;75:180.

[23] Solsona E, Iborra I, Dumont R, et al. The 3-month clinical response to intravesical therapy as a predictive factor for progression in patients with high risk superficial bladder cancer. J Urol 2000;164:685.

[24] Millan-Rodriguez F, Chechile-Toniolo G, Salvador-Bayarri J, et al. Multivariate analysis of the prognostic factors of primary superficial bladder cancer. J Urol 2000;163:73–8.

[25] Pfister C, Flaman JM, Dunet F, et al. p53 mutations in bladder tumors inactivate the transactivation of the p21 and Bax genes, and have a predictive value for the clinical outcome after bacillus Calmette-Guérin therapy. J Urol 1999; 162:69.

[26] Lebret T, Becette V, Barbagelatta M, et al. Correlation between p53 over expression and response to bacillus Calmette-Guérin therapy in a high risk select population of patients with T1G3 bladder cancer. J Urol 1998;159:788.

[27] Lacombe L, Dalbagni G, Zhang ZF, et al. Overexpression of p53 protein in a high risk population of patients with superficial bladder cancer before and

after bacillus Calmette-Guérin therapy: correlation to clinical outcome. J Clin Oncol 1996;14:2646.

[28] Pages F, Flam TA, Vieillefond A, et al. p53 status does not predict initial clinical response to bacillus Calmette-Guérin intravesical therapy in T1 bladder tumors. J Urol 1998;159:1079.

[29] Llopis J, Alcaraz A, Ribal MJ, et al. p53 expression predicts progression and poor survival in T1 bladder tumors. Eur Urol 2000;37:644.

[30] Sarkis AS, Dalbagni G, Cordon-Cardo C, et al. Nuclear overexpression of p53 protein in transitional cell bladder carcinoma: a marker for disease progression. J Natl Cancer Inst 1993;85:53.

[31] Esrig D, Elmajian D, Groshen S, et al. Accumulation of nuclear p53 and tumor progression in bladder cancer. N Engl J Med 1994;331:1259.

[32] Steiner G, Bierhoff E, Schmidt D, et al. p53 immunoreactivity in biopsy specimens of T1G3 transitional cell carcinoma of the bladder: a helpful parameter in guiding the decision for or against cystectomy? Eur J Cancer 2000;36:610.

[33] Lopez-Beltran A, Luque RJ, Alvarez-Kindelan J, et al. Prognostic factors in stage T1 grade 3 bladder cancer survival: the role of G1-S modulators (p53, p21Waf1, p27kip1, cyclin D1, and cyclin D3) and proliferation index (ki67–MIB1). Eur Urol 2004; 45:606–12.

[34] Lamm DL, Blumenstein BA, Crawford ED, et al. Randomized intergroup comparison of bacillus Calmette-Guérin immunotherapy and mitomycin C chemotherapy prophylaxis in superficial transitional cell carcinoma of the bladder. A Southwest Oncology Group Study. Urol Oncol 1995;1:119.

[35] Malmström PU, Wijkström H, Lundholm C, et al. 5-year follow-up of a randomized prospective study comparing mitomycin C and bacillus Calmette-Guérin in patients with superficial bladder carcinoma. Swedish-Norwegian Bladder Cancer Study Group. J Urol 1999;161:1124.

[36] Malmström P. Improved patient outcomes with BCG immunotherapy vs. chemotherapy: Swedish and worldwide experience. Eur Urol Suppl 2000; 37:16.

[37] Zhao W, Schorey JS, Bong-Mastek M, et al. Role of a bacillus Calmette-Guérin fibronectin attachment protein in BCG-induced antitumor activity. Int J Cancer 2000;86:83.

[38] Luo Y, Chen X, Downs TM, et al. INF-alpha 2b enhances Th1 cytokine responses in bladder cancer patients receiving *Mycobacterium bovis* BCG immunotherapy. J Immunol 1999;162:2399.

[39] Bohle A, Thanhauser A, Ulmer AJ, et al. Dissecting the immunobiological effects of bacillus Calmette-Guérin (BCG) in vitro: evidence of a distinct BCG-activated killer (BAK) cell phenomenon. J Urol 1993;150:1932.

[40] Ratliff TL, Haaff EO, Catalona WJ. Interleukin-2 production during intravesical bacille Calmette-

Guérin therapy for bladder cancer. Clin Immunol Immunopathol 1986;40:375.

[41] Cookson MS, Sarosdy MF. Management of stage T1 superficial bladder cancer with intravesical bacillus Calmette-Guérin therapy. J Urol 1992;148: 797.

[42] Brake M, Loertzer H, Horsch R, et al. Recurrence and progression of stage T1, grade 3 transitional cell carcinoma of the bladder following intravesical immunotherapy with bacillus Calmette-Guérin. J Urol 2000;163:1697.

[43] Herr HW. Tumor progression and survival in patients with T1G3 bladder tumours: 15-year outcome. Br J Urol 1997;80:762.

[44] Hurle R, Losa A, Manzetti A, Lembo A. Intravesical bacille Calmette-Guérin in Stage T1 grade 3 bladder cancer therapy: a 7-year follow-up. Urology 1999;54(2):258–63.

[45] Shelley MD, Court JB, Kynaston H, et al. Intravesical bacillus Calmette-Guérin in Ta and T1 bladder cancer (Cochrane Review). Cochrane Database Syst Rev 2000;4:CD001986.

[46] Lamm DL. Bacillus Calmette-Guérin immunotherapy for bladder cancer. J Urol 1985;134:40.

[47] Herr HW, Pinsky CM, Whitmore WF Jr, et al. Experience with intravesical bacillus Calmette-Guérin therapy of superficial bladder tumors. Urology 1985;25:119.

[48] Rubben H, Lutzeyer W, Fischer N, et al. Natural history and treatment of low and high risk superficial bladder tumors. J Urol 1988;139:283.

[49] Melekos MD, Chionis H, Pantazakos A, et al. Intravesical bacillus Calmette-Guérin immunoprophylaxis of superficial bladder cancer: results of a controlled prospective trial with modified treatment schedule. J Urol 1993;149:744.

[50] Smith JA Jr, Labasky RF, Cockett AT, et al. Bladder cancer clinical guidelines panel summary report on the management of nonmuscle invasive bladder cancer (stages Ta, T1 and Tis). American Urological Association. J Urol 1999;162:1697.

[51] Lundholm C, Norlén BJ, Ekman P, et al. A randomized prospective study comparing long-term intravesical instillations of mitomycin C and bacillus Calmette-Guérin in patients with superficial bladder carcinoma. J Urol 1996;156:372.

[52] Brosman SA. Bacillus Calmette-Guérin immunotherapy: techniques and results. Urol Clin North Am 1992;19:557.

[53] Kavoussi LR, Torrence RJ, Gillen DP, et al. Results of 6 weekly intravesical BCG instillations on the treatment of superficial bladder tumors. J Urol 1988;139:935.

[54] Lamm DL, Blumenstein BA, Crissman JD, et al. Maintenance bacillus Calmette-Guérin immunotherapy for recurrent Ta, T1 and carcinoma in situ TCC of the bladder: a randomized Southwest Oncology Group study. J Urol 2000;163: 1124.

[55] Van der Meijden APM, Brausi M, Zambon V, et al. Intravesical instillation of epirubicin, B. C. G., and B. C. G. plus isoniazid for intermediate and high risk Ta, T1 papillary carcinoma of the bladder: a European Organization for Research and Treatment of Cancer Genito-Urinary Group Randomized Phase III trial. J Urol 2001;166:476.

[56] Badalament RA, Farah RN. Treatment of superficial bladder cancer with intravesical chemotherapy. Semin Surg Oncol 1997;13:335.

[57] Sekine H, Fukui I, Yamada T, et al. Intravesical mitomycin C and doxorubicin sequential therapy for carcinoma in situ of the bladder: a longer followup result. J Urol 1994;151:27.

[58] Duque JL, Loughlin KR. An overview of the treatment of superficial bladder cancer: intravesical chemotherapy. Urol Clin North Am 2000;27:125.

[59] Huben RP. Intravesical chemotherapy versus immunotherapy for superficial bladder cancer. Semin Urol Oncol 1996;14:17.

[60] Solsona E, Iborra I, Ricos JV, et al. Effectiveness of a single immediate mitomycin C instillation in patients with low risk superficial bladder cancer: short and low-term followup. J Urol 1999;161:1120.

[61] Isaka S, Okano T, Abe K, et al. Sequential instillation therapy with mitomycin C and Adriamycin for superficial bladder cancer. Cancer Chemother Pharmacol 1992;30:s41.

[62] Fukui I, Kihara K, Sekine H, et al. Intravesical combination chemotherapy with mitomycin C and doxorubicin for superficial bladder cancer: a randomized trial of maintenance versus no maintenance following a complete response. Cancer Chemother Pharmacol 1992;30:37.

[63] Oosterlinck W, Kurth KH, Schroder F, et al. A prospective European Organization for Research and Treatment of Cancer Genitourinary Group randomized trial comparing transurethral resection followed by a single intravesical instillation of epirubicin or water in single stage Ta, T1 papillary carcinoma of the bladder. J Urol 1993;149:749–52.

[64] Tolley DA, Parmar MK, Grigor KM, et al. The effect of intravesical mitomycin C on recurrence of newly diagnosed superficial bladder cancer: a further report with 7 years of follow up. J Urol 1996;155:1233–8.

[65] Solsona E, Iborra I, Ricos JV, et al. Effectiveness of a single immediate mitomycin C instillation in patients with low risk superficial bladder cancer: short and long-term followup. J Urol 1999;161:1120–3.

[66] Bouffioux C, Kurth KH, Bono A, et al. Intravesical adjuvant chemotherapy for superficial transitional cell bladder carcinoma: results of 2 European Organization for Research and Treatment of Cancer randomized trials with mitomycin C and doxorubicin comparing early versus delayed instillations and short-term versus long-term treatment. European Organization for Research and Treatment of Cancer Genitourinary Group. J Urol 1995;153(3 Pt 2):934–41.

[67] Pfister C, Lande P, Herve JM, et al. T1G3 bladder tumors: the respective role of BCG and cystectomy. Prog Urol 1995;5:231–7.

[68] Lebret T, Gaudez F, Herve JM, et al. Low-dose BCG instillations in the treatment of stage T1 grade 3 bladder tumours: recurrence, progression and success. Eur Urol 1998;34:67–72.

[69] Brake M, Loertzer H, Horsch R, et al. Recurrence and progression of stage T1, grade 3 transitional cell carcinoma of the bladder following intravesical immunotherapy with bacillus Calmette-Guérin. J Urol 2000;163:1697–701.

[70] Patard JJ, Moudouni S, Saint F, et al. Tumor progression and survival in patients with T1G3 bladder tumors: multicentric retrospective study comparing 94 patients treated during 17 years. Urology 2001;58:551–6.

[71] Kulkarni JN, Gupta R. Recurrence and progression in stage T1G3 bladder tumour with intravesical bacille Calmette-Guérin Danish 1331 strain. BJU Int 2002;90:554–7.

[72] Bogdanovic J, Marusic G, Djozic J, et al. The management of T1G3 bladder cancer. Urol Int 2002;69:263–5.

[73] Peyromaure M, Guerin F, Amsellem-Ouazana D, et al. Intravesical bacillus Calmette-Guérin therapy for stage T1 grade 3 transitional cell carcinoma of the bladder: recurrence, progression and survival in a study of 57 patients. J Urol 2003;169:2110–2.

[74] Shahin O, Thalmann GN, Rentsch C, et al. A retrospective analysis of 153 patients treated with or without intravesical bacillus Calmette-Guérin for primary stage T1 grade 3 bladder cancer: recurrence, progression and survival. J Urol 2003;169:96–100.

[75] Herr HW, Dalbagni G. Defining bacillus Calmette-Guérin refractory superficial bladder tumors. J Urol 2003;169:1706–8.

[76] Pansadoro V, Emiliozzi P, De Paula F, et al. Long-term follow-up of G3T1 transitional cell carcinoma of the bladder treated with intravesical bacille Calmette-Guérin: 18-year experience. Urology 2002;59:227–31.

[77] Malmstrom PU, Wijkstrom H, Lundholm C, et al. 5-year followup of a randomized prospective study comparing mitomycin C and bacillus Calmette-Guérin in patients with superficial bladder carcinoma. Swedish-Norwegian Bladder Cancer Study Group. J Urol 1999;161:1124–7.

[78] Steinberg G, Bahnson R, Brosman S, et al. Efficacy and safety of valrubicin for the treatment of bacillus Calmette-Guérin refractory carcinoma in situ of the bladder. J Urol 2000;163:761–7.

[79] Belldegrun AS, Franklin JR, O'Donnell MA, et al. Superficial bladder cancer: the role of interferon-alpha. J Urol 1998;159:1793–801.

[80] Punnen SP, Chin JL, Jewett MA. Management of bacillus Calmette-Guérin (BCG) refractory superficial bladder cancer: results with intravesical BCG and interferon combination therapy. Can J Urol 2003;10:1790–5.

[81] Lam JS, Benson MC, O'Donnell MA, et al. Bacillus Calmette-Guérin plus interferon-alpha2B intravesical therapy maintains an extended treatment plan for superficial bladder cancer with minimal toxicity. Urol Oncol 2003;21:354–60.

[82] O'Donnell MA, Lilli K, Leopold C. Interim results from a national multicenter phase II trial of combination bacillus Calmette-Guérin plus interferon alfa-2B for superficial bladder cancer. J Urol 2004;176:888–92.

[83] Dunst J, Sauer R, Schrott KM, et al. Organ-sparing treatment of advanced bladder cancer: a 10-year experience. Int J Radiat Oncol Biol Phys 1994;30: 261–6.

[84] Rodel C, Dunst J, Grabenbauer GG, et al. Radiotherapy is an effective treatment for high-risk T1-bladder cancer. Strahlenther Onkol 2001;177: 82–8.

[85] Berger AP, Steiner H, Stenzl A, et al. Photodynamic therapy with intravesical instillation of 5-aminolevulinic acid for patients with recurrent superficial bladder cancer: a single center study. Urology 2003;61:338–41.

[86] Cookson MS, Herr HW, Zhang ZF, et al. The treated natural history of high risk superficial bladder cancer: 15-year outcome. J Urol 1997;158:62.

[87] Malkowicz BS, Nichols P, Lieskovsky G, et al. The role of radical cystectomy in the management of high grade superficial bladder cancer (PA, PI, PIS and P2). J Urol 1990;144:641.

[88] Malavaud B. T1G3 bladder tumours: the case for radical cystectomy. Eur Urol 2004;45:406–10.

[89] Herr HW. A retrospective analysis of 153 patients treated with or without intravesical bacillus Calmette-Guérin for primary stage T1 grade 3 bladder cancer: recurrence, progression and survival [editorial comment]. J Urol 2003;169:96–100.

[90] Dyrskjot L, Thykjaer T, Kruhoffer M, et al. Identifying distinct classes of bladder carcinoma using microarrays. Nat Genet 2003;33:90–6.

[91] Herr HW, Sogani PC. Does early cystectomy improve the survival of patients with high risk superficial bladder tumors? J Urol 2001;166: 1296–9.

[92] Hart S, Skinner EC, Meyerowitz BE, et al. Quality of life after radical cystectomy for bladder cancer in patients with an ileal conduit, cutaneous or urethral Kock pouch. J Urol 1999;162:77–81.

[93] Henningsohn L, Steven K, Kallestrup EB, et al. Distressful symptoms and well-being after radical cystectomy and orthotopic bladder substitution compared with a matched control population. J Urol 2002;168:168–74.

[94] Hautman RE, dePetriconi R, Gottfried HW, et al. The ileal neobladder: complications and functional results in 363 patients after 11 years of followup. J Urol 1999;161:422.

[95] Soloway MS, Sofer M, Vaidya A. Contemporary management of stage T1 transitional cell carcinoma of the bladder. J Urol 2002;167:1573–83.

[96] Rintala E, Jauhiainen K, Kaasinene E, et al. Alternating mitomycin C and bacillus Calmette-Guérin instillation prophylaxis for recurrent papillary (stages Ta to T1) superficial bladder cancer. Finnbladder Group. J Urol 1996;156:56.

[97] Witjes JA, Caris CT, Mungan NA, et al. Results of a randomized phase III trial of sequential intravesical therapy with mitomycin C and bacillus Calmette-Guérin versus mitomycin C alone in patients with superficial bladder cancer. J Urol 1998;160:1668.

[98] Ali-El-Dein B, Nabeeh A, Ismail EH, et al. Sequential bacillus Calmette-Guérin and epirubicin versus bacillus Calmette-Guérin alone for superficial bladder tumors: a randomized prospective study. J Urol 1999;162:339.

[99] Bilen CY, Ozen H, Aki FT, et al. Clinical experience with BCG alone versus BCG plus epirubicin. Int J Urol 2000;7:206.

[100] Bono AV, Lovisolo JA, Saredi G. Transurethral resection and sequential chemo-immunoprophylaxis in primary T1G3 bladder cancer. Eur Urol 2000; 37:478.

[101] Serretta V, Pavone C, Ingargiola GB, et al. TUR and adjuvant intravesical chemotherapy in T1G3 bladder tumors: recurrence, progression and survival in 137 selected patients followed up to 20 years. Eur Urol 2004;45:730–5.

[102] Dalbagni G, Russo P, Sheinfeld J, et al. Phase I trial of intravesical gemcitabine in bacillus Calmette-Guerin-refractory transitional-cell carcinoma of the bladder [see comment]. J Clin Oncol 2002;20: 3193–8.

[103] Dalbagni G, Mazumdar M, Russo P, et al. Phase II trial of intravesical gemcitabine in BCG-refractory transitional cell carcinoma of the bladder. J Urol 2004;171(4)(Suppl):72 (abstract).

[104] Laufer M, Ramalingam S, Schoenberg MP, et al. Intravesical gemcitabine therapy for superficial transitional cell carcinoma of the bladder: a phase I and pharmacokinetic study. J Clin Oncol 2003; 21:697–703.

[105] De Berardinis E, Antonini G, Peters GJ, et al. Intravesical administration of gemcitabine in superficial bladder cancer: a phase I study with pharmacodynamic evaluation. BJU Int 2004;93: 491–4.

[106] Au JL, Kalns J, Gan Y, et al. Pharmacologic effects of paclitaxel in human bladder tumors. Cancer Chemother Pharmacol 1997;41:69–74.

[107] Chen D, Song D, Wientjes MG, et al. Effect of dimethyl sulfoxide on bladder tissue penetration of inravesical paclitaxel. Clin Cancer Res 2003;9: 363–9.

[108] Gomella LG, Mastrangelo MJ, McCue PA, et al. Phase I study of intravesical vaccinia virus as a vector for gene therapy of bladder cancer. J Urol 2001; 166:1291–5.

[109] Morales A, Voccia I, Steinhoff G, et al. Mycobacterium phlei cell wall extract for the treatment of superficial bladder cancer: final results of a phase 2 trial. J Urol 2004;171:74.

[110] Doll RJ, Kirschmeier P, Bishop WR. Farnesyl-transferase inhibitors as anticancer agents. Curr Opin Drug Discov Dev 2004;7:478–86.

[111] Thiounn N, Pages F, Mejean A, et al. Adoptive immunotherapy for superficial bladder cancer with autologous macrophage activated killer cells. J Urol 2002;168:2373–6.

[112] Colombo R, Da Pozzo LF, Salonia A, et al. Multicentric study comparing intravesical chemotherapy alone and with local microwave hyperthermia for prophylaxis of recurrence of superficial transitional cell carcinoma. J Clin Oncol 2003;21: 4270–6.

[113] Di Stasi SM, Giannantoni A, Stephen RL, et al. Intravesical electromotive mitomycin C versus passive transport mitomycin C for high risk superficial bladder cancer: a prospective randomized study. J Urol 2003;170:777–82.

ELSEVIER
SAUNDERS

Urol Clin N Am 32 (2005) 147–155

UROLOGIC
CLINICS
of North America

Radical Cystectomy for Bladder Cancer: The Case for Early Intervention

Sam S. Chang, MD*, Michael S. Cookson, MD

*Department of Urologic Surgery, Vanderbilt University Medical Center,
A-1302 Medical Center North, Nashville, TN 37232-2765, USA*

Approximately 20% of patients with bladder cancer are found to harbor invasive disease at presentation. Radical cystectomy remains the gold standard for patients with muscle invasive urothelial carcinoma of the bladder and is an important option for patients with high-grade non–muscle invasive disease, including those who have recurrent disease after intravesical therapy or disease refractory to attempted conservative therapy [1]. In fact, as many as one third of contemporary cystectomies are performed among patients with clinical stage Ta/T1 or carcinoma in situ (CIS). Most of these patients have tumor characteristics that would be considered high risk for disease progression, and many have previously undergone multiple failed attempts at bladder preservation, providing ample justification for exenterative surgery.

In the decision process, most of these patients are offered what some would consider an "early cystectomy," because they are believed to have non–muscle invasive tumors. Unfortunately, pathologic staging at the time of cystectomy indicates that 35% to 50% of these patients, in fact, harbor muscle invasive disease, including micrometastases in 10% to 15%. In addition, patient outcomes seem to be directly related to the pathologic stage, implying an adverse effect owing to a delay in treatment [2]. Despite the intent to perform early cystectomy, the reality remains that for an unacceptably high percentage of these patients, this notion is, in fact, a misreckoning.

The concept of early or perhaps better-described "timely" cystectomy can be extended further to patients with muscle invasive disease. Improvements in surgical technique and perioperative care have led to decreased mortality and morbidity rates [3]. Despite these improvements and the use of orthotopic urinary diversion, many patients do not proceed quickly to radical cystectomy for different reasons. These reasons include the time needed for the completion of a metastatic evaluation and preoperative medical preparation, physician scheduling delays, patient comorbidities, the time taken by patients seeking multiple opinions, the initiation of neoadjuvant therapies such as radiation or chemotherapy, and socioeconomic issues, among others. Although it is prudent to evaluate patients thoroughly and to assess perioperative risk in preparation for radical cystectomy, unnecessary delays can have adverse consequences. Increasingly, reports of the negative impact of a delay in cystectomy on pathologic staging are emerging [4,5]. Furthermore, delaying cystectomy in patients with invasive disease has been associated with a decrease in disease-specific survival [6,7].

Herein, the authors review the status of early cystectomy in different settings with an emphasis on strategies design to align this concept with its intention to reduce deaths among patients with this potentially lethal disease.

Early radical cystectomy in noninvasive disease: indicators of high-risk superficial disease

Although most superficial bladder cancer is treated safely and effectively by transurethral resection or intravesical therapies, some forms of non–muscle invasive transitional cell carcinoma

---

* Corresponding author.
E-mail address: sam.chang@vanderbilt.edu
(S.S. Chang).

0094-0143/05/$ - see front matter © 2005 Elsevier Inc. All rights reserved.
doi:10.1016/j.ucl.2005.01.001

have a high propensity to invade. Although it remains impossible to predict accurately which tumors will progress or may have already progressed, there are certain prognostic factors that the urologist should take into account.

Chromosomal alterations and cell cycle regulators

An abnormal number of chromosomes and chromosomes of abnormal morphology have been associated with an increased risk of bladder cancer recurrence and progression [8,9]. Several studies correlate polysomy, especially of chromosome 7, or aneuploidy with progression of superficial bladder cancer [10–12].

Alterations in chromosomes encoding 17p, p53, p21, and pRb have been thought to influence the likelihood of progression and survival in patients with invasive and superficial disease. Recently, experience at the University of Southern California (USC) has demonstrated that an alteration of three proteins (p53, p21, pRb) provides more information than a single alteration. Each one of these alterations was an independent predictor of disease recurrence and overall survival, but the combination of all three provided the most information [13]. As individual determinants, the p53, p21, and pRb status were independent predictors of the time to recurrence ($P < .001$, $P < .001$, and $P < .001$, respectively) and overall survival ($P < .001$, $P = .002$, and $P = .001$, respectively). The 5-year recurrence rate was 23% in patients without any alterations and increased as more protein alterations were found. The rate was 32% for a single alteration, 57% for two alterations, and 93% for all three alterations (log-rank, $P < .001$). Similarly, the 5-year survival rates corresponded with the number of alterations, with a rate of 70% for no alterations, 58% for one alteration, 33% for two alterations, and 8% for all three alterations, respectively (log-rank, $P < .001$). After stratifying by stage, the number of altered proteins remained significantly associated with the time to recurrence and overall survival [13].

Another oncogene suggested as a useful prognostic marker for bladder cancer is erbB-2. This oncogene encodes a growth factor receptor that is functionally related to epidermal growth factor receptor. Its amplification and overexpression have been found to correlate with recurrence in patients who have superficial bladder tumors [14].

Despite shortcomings, the combination of the clinical findings of grade, stage, and CIS represent the most important risk factors in superficial disease [15].

High-grade disease

The combination of tumor grade and the depth of invasion continues to be the most commonly used and helpful predictor of bladder cancer behavior and progression [16]. This observation is especially true in patients with superficial disease. Patients with superficial grade 1 and 2 tumors have approximately a 10% risk for muscle invasion, whereas one third of patients with grade 3 tumors will eventually have invasive disease [17]. Well-differentiated tumors, in fact, are fundamentally different from high-grade tumors, and these genetic differences may explain the different behavior of these tumors [18].

Carcinoma in situ

The presence of CIS increases the likelihood of more advanced disease or the development of advanced disease. Among patients thought to have CIS or disease confined to the urothelium, as many as 20% who are treated with cystectomy are found to contain some elements of microscopic invasion [19]. Between 40% and 83% of CIS tumors will ultimately progress to muscle invasion [20]. In a recent series examining patients with high-grade T1 bladder cancer, Masood et al [21] demonstrated that the presence of CIS led to an upstaging of lesions in 55% of radical cystectomy specimens as opposed to 6% in bladders without CIS.

Tumor stage

The depth of invasion even in superficial disease may predict the likelihood of tumor progression. In one series, progression was seen in 5% of lesions that had only superficial lamina propria invasion as opposed to almost 50% progression in patients who had deeper lamina propria involvement of the muscularis mucosa [22]. The importance of stage has been validated by the efforts of uropathologists to delineate T1 classification because of its possible impact on tumor recurrence and progression [23]. Although cystectomy is clearly indicated in patients with uncontrollable Ta disease or intravesical therapy–refractory CIS, the decision and the timing to proceeding to cystectomy may be most crucial and most difficult in patients with T1 disease and other high-risk features.

Early radical cystectomy in noninvasive disease: T1 tumors

Urothelial tumors that invade the lamina propria but not the muscularis propria are a particularly problematic clinical entity. One of seemingly easy but often difficult initial steps is ensuring that the tumor has been completely resected. Ensuring that the tumor does not invade the bladder muscle is the joint responsibility of the surgeon, who must provide adequate muscle in the specimen, and the pathologist, who must note the presence or absence of muscle involvement. Indeed, many times clinical understaging remains the "Achilles' heel" of T1 tumor treatment. Increasing uncertainty is the fact that the tumor biology of T1 tumors is unpredictable, with the rate of stage progression ranging from 15% to 50%.

Prognostic and practical aspects of the depth of invasion

In an attempt to differentiate among these tumors, it has been proposed that the depth of lamina propria invasion may be an important prognostic indicator [24]. In one series, stratification by into two groups, those with (pT1b) or without cancer invasion to or near the muscularis mucosae (pT1a), resulted in significantly different progression rates of 53.5% and 6.7%, respectively [22]. In another series, the 5-year progression-free survival rate of 67% for patients with a depth of invasion of $\geq$ 1.5 mm was less than the 93% survival rate for patients with a depth of invasion of $\leq$ 1.5 mm [24]. Other investigators, including Platz et al [25], have found no difference in 10-year survival rates in patients with invasion above the muscularis mucosae (65%) and patients with invasion below the muscularis mucosae (60%).

One of the inherent difficulties in substaging these tumors remains the pathologic artifact created by transurethral resection and the lack of orientation. In addition, the muscularis mucosae may be identifiable in only half of specimens. Accordingly, the 1998 Bladder Consensus Conference Committee concluded that "substage based on the relationship of tumor to muscularis mucosae should not be universally adopted or advocated by pathologist" [26]. Nevertheless, they recommended that pathologists should be encouraged to provide some assessment as to the extent of lamina propria invasion (ie, focal versus extensive) to help guide urologists in patient management. Despite its potential, for the foreseeable future, the added benefit of reporting the depth of invasion among T1 tumors will be dependent on the experience and diligence of the pathologist and most likely will not be widely available to the practicing clinician.

Problem of clinical understaging

The accuracy of clinical staging is of particular importance when major differences in treatment that may directly impact patient outcome exist based on subtle differences in pathology. With respect to noninvasive tumors, clinical understaging is particularly problematic, with staging errors ranging from 27% to 62% (Table 1) [27–35]. This error is due in part to the limitations is radiographic imaging, which are known to understage bladder cancer even in patients with known muscle invasive disease [36,37]. The most important factor in noninvasive bladder cancer is meticulous pathologic assessment of the transurethral resection specimen.

In one series, Dutta et al reported that the rate of clinical understaging was 46% among patients with clinical T1 tumors who underwent radical cystectomy [27]. Grade was not predictive of understaging; however, the presence of uninvolved muscularis propria in the transurethral resection specimen was a significant predictor of understaging (P = 0.01). Of the 63 patients with stage T1 disease, 41% had no muscularis propria in the transurethral resection specimen. Among these cases, 62% were understaged. On the other hand, only 30% of patients with stage T1 disease and uninvolved muscularis propria in the transurethral resection specimen were understaged; therefore, the presence of uninvolved muscularis propria significantly reduces but does not eliminate the risk of clinical understaging. Perhaps most notably, understaging was associated with

Table 1
Understaging in T1 disease

Study	Year	Patients understaged (%)
Pagano et al [31]	1991	35
Amling et al [29]	1994	37
Soloway et al [32]	1994	36
Freeman et al [34]	1995	34
Ghoneim et al [33]	1997	62
Stein et al [61]	2000	39
Dutta et al [27]	2001	40
Bianco et al [35]	2004	27

statistically worse disease-specific and recurrence-free survival, supporting early observations of the negative impact of understaging on survival [34]. These findings provide a backdrop for arguments in favor of improved methods of detection and refinements in pathologic staging.

Role of repeat transurethral resection

Owing to limitations in clinical staging, it has been proposed that one offer patients with clinical stage T1 tumors a repeat transurethral resection within the first 4 to 6 weeks of initial resection. The stated goals include the verification of complete tumor resection, an assessment for evidence of multifocality or associated CIS, and an attempt to reduce the rate of understaging. These goals are of particular importance when muscularis propria is not present in the initial specimen. In a review, Miladi et al [38] found that a second transurethral resection performed within 6 weeks of the initial resection detected residual tumor in 26% to 83% of cases. More importantly, it may correct clinical staging errors in as many as 49% of cases and is particularly warranted for T1 tumors requiring a change in management.

Herr [39] reported the results in 150 cases involving repeat transurethral resection. In this series, 76% of patients had residual tumor on repeat transurethral resection. Of 96 cases with superficial (Ta, Tis, T1) bladder tumors, 75% had residual noninvasive tumor, and 29% were upstaged to invasive tumor. Furthermore, the results of the second transurethral resection changed treatment in 50 patients (33%). In another series, Grimm et al [40] reported the results of repeat transurethral resection in 124 patients with noninvasive tumors. Residual tumor was found in 33% of all repeat transurethral resections, including 27% of patients with Ta tumors and 53% with T1 disease. Of those tumors, 81% were located at the initial tumor resection site. Rigaud et al [41] reported the results of repeat resection in 52 patients with a first diagnosis of T1 bladder tumor. Of the 52 patients, 19 (36.5%) had residual disease on the second transurethral resection. Residual tumor was revealed at the initial resection site in 84.2% of cases and was significantly more frequently found in patients with multifocal tumors than in patients with solitary tumors (58% versus 24%). It was concluded that a second endoscopic procedure was essential to ensure the absence of residual tumor before starting conservative treatment for T1 bladder tumors.

These data support the role of repeat transurethral resection among patients with high-risk noninvasive urothelial carcinoma. It is recommended that this repeat transurethral resection be performed within 6 weeks of the initial resection, and that the strategy include resection of the initial tumor bed as well as random or directed biopsies to assess for multifocality or CIS. Patients whose specimens do not contain identifiable muscularis propria and those with multifocal tumors seem to be at highest risk for residual disease. The presence of muscle invasion on repeat resection should identify patients in whom a change in treatment strategy should be considered. Furthermore, the response to bladder-conserving strategies including intravesical therapy is likely to be enhanced following complete tumor resection.

Indications for radical cystectomy in patients with T1 tumors

The natural history of treated patients with high-risk non–muscle invasive disease has been examined. Among patients with CIS, the death rate from bladder cancer at 10 years may be as high as 20% [42]. In addition, among patients with noninvasive tumors treated with initial intravesical therapy, progression rates as high as 53% have been observed, with death from bladder cancer occurring in as many as one-third of those followed for up to 15 years [43]. Some patients with non–muscle invasive disease harbor potentially lethal tumors justifying aggressive surgical intervention when clinically indicated.

The inherent difficulty is the fact that predicting tumor biology remains largely an art rather than science, with significant room for subjective clinical interpretation. The indications for radical cystectomy among patients with noninvasive disease include high-grade disease recurrence after intravesical therapy. Patients with stage T1 tumors, including those with associated CIS, are at particular risk for progression. Patients with CIS refractory to conservative intravesical therapy including salvage therapy should also be offered the option of radical cystectomy [44]. Currently, despite high-risk features, most patients are offered initial management with the goal of bladder preservation. This treatment usually includes at least one course of intravesical therapy following initial transurethral resection. Strong consideration should be given to repeat resection among patients with stage T1 tumors, and repeat biopsies following intravesical therapy are particularly important among patients treated for CIS. Some patients may choose cystectomy as an initial treatment option, which must be balanced against the potential risks, benefits, and impact on quality of life.

Outcome of radical cystectomy in noninvasive disease

The long-term benefit of radical cystectomy is excellent among patients in whom the cancer has not yet invaded muscle. In a recent series of T1 tumors treated with cystectomy, the estimated 10-year disease-free survival rate for pathologic T1 tumors was 92% [35]. This rate was compared with a 64% 10-year disease-free survival among those with muscle invasion at the time of cystectomy. Similar excellent survival rates have been reported in many series [27,29,33,34,45]. In a large cohort from USC with long-term follow-up, the 10-year recurrence-free survival rate among patients with pathologic T1 tumors was 78% [46].

The previously mentioned reports document excellent long-term survival for the majority of patients with non–muscle invasive disease treated with radical cystectomy. This outcome is most likely in patients without metastatic disease. This observation has called into question the timing of radical cystectomy and its impact on patient outcome. Stockle et al [47] reported survival rates among patients based on the timing of cystectomy. Among those with T1 tumors, the 5-year recurrence-free survival rate in the immediate cystectomy group was 90% compared with 62% in the delayed group. These data from more than a decade ago support the concept of improved survival with early cystectomy.

In a subsequent study, Herr and Sogani compared survival after early versus delayed cystectomy among patients with high-risk non-invasive bladder tumors. Of 307 patients treated initially with transurethral resection and bacillus Calmette-Guerin (BCG) therapy, 90 (29%) underwent cystectomy for recurrent tumor. For 35 patients with recurrent noninvasive tumors, the survival rate was 92% when the cystectomy was performed within 2 years of initial BCG therapy compared with 56% in patients who underwent cystectomy more than 2 years after initial BCG therapy. The issue of timing was similarly pronounced among 55 patients with recurrent muscle invasive bladder disease; 41% and 18% of patients survived when cystectomy was performed within and after 2 years, respectively. Multivariate analysis showed that survival was improved in patients who underwent earlier rather than delayed cystectomy for non–muscle invasive tumor relapse. It was concluded that earlier cystectomy improves the long-term survival of patients with high-risk superficial bladder tumors in whom BCG therapy fails [2].

The impact of radical cystectomy on the quality of life of patients with non–muscle invasive bladder cancer should be weighed in the decision when considering treatment options. Some have suggested that the ability to offer orthotopic diversion may reduce physician reluctance to offer cystectomy and may have a positive influence on the timing of surgery. In one series of 213 men with invasive bladder cancer, patients were evaluated from the interval of primary diagnosis to cystectomy, as well as the number of previous transurethral resections before cystectomy [48]. A total of 135 patients underwent an ileal neobladder and 78 a conduit diversion. In the neobladder and conduit groups, an average of 2.1 and 4.1 transurethral resections were performed, respectively. The interval from the primary diagnosis to cystectomy was 11.8 months in the neobladder group and 16.7 months in the conduit group. Cystectomy was performed 4.1 months after the diagnosis of invasive cancer in the neobladder group, whereas cystectomy was delayed for 15.4 months in the conduit group. Cancer-specific 5-year survival rates were 76.6% and 28.35% in the neobladder and conduit groups, respectively. After stratifying according to tumor stage, the 5-year survival rate was significantly higher for all disease stages in the neobladder group when compared with the conduit group. These data suggest that the ileal neobladder may decrease physician reluctance to perform cystectomy early in the disease process, increasing the survival rate. They also demonstrate that the ileal neobladder option prompts an earlier patient and physician decision in favor of cystectomy.

Although these studies have limitations given their retrospective methodology and selection bias, the impact of timing on the outcome of cystectomy seems to be significant. More importantly, it is a variable that clinicians can influence and should include in the counseling of patients with high-risk non–muscle invasive disease. These findings suggest that cystectomy should be offered to patients at high risk in a more timely fashion than what has been offered historically. Certainly, improvements in perioperative management have reduced the morbidity and mortality associated with contemporary cystectomy [49]. The potential for improvements in quality of life afforded with continent orthotopic urinary diversion and nerve-sparing radical cystectomy are attractive options for young highly motivated patients confronted with a potentially lethal, yet currently organ-confined disease.

Radical cystectomy in invasive disease

Patients who are diagnosed with muscle invasive bladder cancer are a diverse population who require careful evaluation and staging before determining the best treatment option. Although other viable options exist for high-risk superficial cancer other than early radical cystectomy, surgical removal of the bladder remains the gold standard for muscle invasive cancer. In this group, early or perhaps more aptly labeled "timely" cystectomy is important for the patient's well being. Except for patients with bulky and extensive local disease or bulky lymphadenopathy, as is true in patients with T1 disease, contemporary preoperative evaluation continues to understage patients with invasive transitional cell carcinoma.

Although appropriate time should be given for the consideration of options and pretreatment evaluation, an undue delay may compromise cancer control. The rationale for delaying cystectomy because the patient is "too sick" is becoming increasingly difficult to defend. The morbidity of cystectomy has declined during the last 20 years [50–52]. The authors' data have demonstrated the safety and effectiveness of this procedure even in elderly patients with significant comorbidities [52,53]. Multiple reasons for delay can be patient driven, such as seeking other medical opinions and patient preference. Regardless of the etiology, prolonging the decision algorithm to proceed with cystectomy may prove harmful.

Several studies have supported the negative impact of a delay in cystectomy. In a recent series from the authors' center, over a 4-year period of more than 300 radical cystectomies, 153 patients had muscle invasive disease at diagnosis. Disturbingly, only 44% of these patients had organ-confined disease, and 38% had lymph node involvement. These findings confirm the inherently logical principle that the longer a malignant

disease process has to progress, the more likely the malignancy will grow and advance in stage. Multiple variables can affect tumor pathology, but a statistically significant correlation exists between the time of diagnosis and cystectomy and final pathologic stage. Patients with a greater than 90-day lag between transurethral resection diagnosis and cystectomy were more likely to have pT3 non–organ-confined disease or greater when compared with patients undergoing cystectomy before 90 days (81% versus 52%; $P = 0.01$, chi-square analysis). Age and gender did not correlate with pathologic stage ($P = 0.48$ and 0.49, respectively). Patients with organ-confined disease at the time of radical cystectomy had a mean interval time from diagnosis by transurethral resection of bladder tumor until cystectomy of 47.5 days versus 75.1 days for patients in whom the cystectomy specimen had non–organ-confined disease ($P = 0.02$, t-test). More than 80% of patients in whom radical cystectomy was delayed more than 90 days from the time of transurethral resection diagnosis of muscle invasive disease had advanced, non–organ-confined disease [54].

Additionally, the time from the onset of symptoms until diagnosis and treatment of muscle invasive disease may influence the pathologic stage and, in fact, may be the most predictive of outcome [55]. Hara et al [56] demonstrated a significantly higher proportion of cystectomy specimens with lymphovascular invasion when cystectomy was delayed (73% versus 46%, $P < .05$). Although there was no difference in precystectomy biopsy clinicopathologic characteristics, the patients who underwent removal of the bladder within a 3-month period had a significantly longer recurrence-free, cause-specific, and overall survival rate ($P < .05$ for all comparisons). In fact, the recurrence-free survival was 87% versus 53% when cystectomy was performed within 3 months. Although multiple tumor characteristics were similar, such as size, multiplicity, grade, stage, and nodal stage at cystectomy, the patients in the delayed group were older (72.5 years versus 64.2 years, $P < .01$), and this advanced age may be one of the reasons for a delay.

A review from Memorial Sloan-Kettering Cancer Center demonstrated improved outcomes when cystectomy was performed sooner versus later. The median time from diagnosis until cystectomy was 67 days, and patients' outcomes were better when radical cystectomy was performed within 3 months of diagnosis versus later [57]. Recently, data from the University of

Pennsylvania confirmed these findings for similar time frames. For all patients, the mean interval from diagnosis to cystectomy was 7.9 weeks (range, 1 to 40). Extravesical disease (P3a or greater) or positive nodes were identified in 84% (16 of 19) of patients when the delay was longer than 12 weeks in comparison with 48.2% of patients (82 of 170) with a time lag of 12 weeks or less ($P < .01$). Three-year survival was lower ($34.9\% \pm 13.5\%$) for patients with a surgery delay longer than 12 weeks when compared with those with a shorter interval ($62.1\% \pm 4.5\%$; hazards ratio, 2.51; 95% confidence interval [CI], 1.30–4.83; $P = .006$). When adjusted for nodal status and clinical and pathologic stages, the interval until cystectomy was still statistically significant (adjusted hazards ratio, 1.93; 95% CI, 0.99–3.76; $P = .05$) [6].

The goal of proceeding in a timely fashion is to act before the development of local or distant metastases. Clearly, patients with more advanced disease do worse. In the USC series, patients with non–organ-confined bladder cancer (P3b, P4) and lymph node–negative cancer demonstrated a significantly higher probability of recurrence and death when compared with patients with organ-confined disease [46].

Outcome of radical cystectomy in invasive disease

Radical cystectomy in patients with invasive bladder cancer provides local control and survival benefit [33,58,59]. Long-term survival is best among those with organ-confined disease, and, consistently, 5-year survival is greater than 70% [31,46,60]. In the largest contemporary series to date, investigators at USC reported the results in 1054 patients with a median follow-up of 10.2 years [46]. In that series, the overall recurrence-free survival rates at 5 and 10 years were 68% and 66%, respectively. Patients with muscle invasive disease (P2a and P3a) and lymph node–negative tumors had an 89% and 87% and 78% and 76% 5- and 10-year recurrence-free survival, respectively.

Summary

There are no prospective studies comparing early cystectomy versus cystectomy after failed conservative management in patients with high-risk superficial bladder cancer. In the absence of clinically proven biomarkers for predicting tumor biology and the response to therapy, the treatment decision must be individualized based on the high-risk features outlined herein. Assuming that all patients can be treated effectively with bladder-sparing regimens and safely salvaged at the time of failure or progression is dangerous. Data support the negative impact of a delay in cystectomy and argue for improvements in the timing of cystectomy despite the clinical absence of muscle invasion. Accordingly, high-risk patients with non–muscle invasive disease require vigilant follow-up and should be informed from the onset of the risk for progression and the possible need for cystectomy. Repeat resection before intravesical therapy in the patient with T1 tumor is advised and should help to improve, but will not completely eliminate, the problem of clinical understaging. Among patients with CIS and recurrent high-grade non–muscle invasive tumors, repeat biopsies following intravesical therapy are encouraged to ensure treatment response.

Although there is debate regarding the timing of early cystectomy for patients with high-risk non–muscle invasive bladder cancer, there is little doubt that, for muscle invasive disease, prompt cystectomy influences the effectiveness of this therapy choice. An unnecessary delay in the performance of radical cystectomy in patients with organ-confined bladder cancer compromises outcomes and risks potentially avoidable deaths from disease.

References

[1] Smith JA Jr, Labasky RF, Cockett AT, et al. Bladder cancer clinical guidelines panel summary report on the management of nonmuscle invasive bladder cancer (stages Ta, T1 and TIS): the American Urological Association. J Urol 1999;162(5):1697–701.

[2] Herr HW, Sogani PC. Does early cystectomy improve the survival of patients with high risk superficial bladder tumors? J Urol 2001;166(4):1296–9.

[3] Thrasher JB, Crawford ED. Current management of invasive and metastatic transitional cell carcinoma of the bladder. J Urol 1993;149(5):957–72.

[4] Chang SS, Hassan JM, Cookson M, et al. Delaying radical cystectomy for muscle invasive bladder cancer results in worse pathologic stage. J Urol, in press.

[5] Malkowicz SB, Nichols P, Lieskovsky G, et al. The role of radical cystectomy in the management of high-grade superficial bladder cancer. J Urol 1990; 44:641–5.

[6] Sanchez-Ortiz RF, Huang WC, Mick R, et al. An interval longer than 12 weeks between the diagnosis of muscle invasion and cystectomy is associated with

worse outcome in bladder carcinoma. J Urol 2003; 169(1):110–5; discussion, 115.

[7] Liedberg F, Anderson H, Mansson A, et al. Diagnostic delay and prognosis in invasive bladder cancer. Scand J Urol Nephrol 2003;37(5):396–400.

[8] Falor WH, Ward-Skinner RM. The importance of marker chromosomes in superficial transitional cell carcinoma of the bladder: 50 patients followed up to 17 years. J Urol 1988;139(5):929–32.

[9] Sandberg AA. Chromosome changes in bladder cancer: clinical and other correlations. Cancer Genet Cytogenet 1986;19(1–2):163–75.

[10] Waldman FM, Carroll PR, Kerschmann R, et al. Centromeric copy number of chromosome 7 is strongly correlated with tumor grade and labeling index in human bladder cancer. Cancer Res 1991; 51(14):3807–13.

[11] Watters AD, Going JJ, Grigor KM, et al. Progression to detrusor-muscle invasion in bladder carcinoma is associated with polysomy of chromosomes 1 and 8 in recurrent pTa/pT1 tumours. Eur J Cancer 2002;38(12):1593–9.

[12] Richter J, Wagner U, Schraml P, et al. Chromosomal imbalances are associated with a high risk of progression in early invasive (pT1) urinary bladder cancer. Cancer Res 1999;59(22):5687–91.

[13] Chatterjee SJ, Datar R, Youssefzadeh D, et al. Combined effects of p53, p21, and pRb expression in the progression of bladder transitional cell carcinoma. J Clin Oncol 2004;22(6):1007–13.

[14] Sauter G, Moch H, Moore D, et al. Heterogeneity of erbB-2 gene amplification in bladder cancer. Cancer Res 1993;53(10 Suppl):2199–203.

[15] Millan-Rodriquez F, Chechile-Tomiolo G, Salvador-Bayarri J, et al. Multivariate analysis of the prognostic factors of primary superficial bladder cancer. J Urol 2000;163:73–80.

[16] Stein JP. Indications for early cystectomy. Urology 2003;62(4):591–5.

[17] Torti FM, Lum BL, Aston D, et al. Superficial bladder cancer: the primacy of grade in the development of invasive disease. J Clin Oncol 1987;5(1):125–30.

[18] Cote R, Chatterjee SJ. Molecular determinants of outcome in bladder cancer. Cancer J Sci Am 1999; 5:1–15.

[19] Farrow GM, Utz DC, Rife CC. Morphological and clinical observations of patients with early bladder cancer treated with total cystectomy. Cancer Res 1976;36(7 Pt 2):2495–501.

[20] Althausen AF, Prout GR Jr, Daly JJ. Non-invasive papillary carcinoma of the bladder associated with carcinoma in situ. J Urol 1976;116(5):575–80.

[21] Masood S, Sriprasad S, Palmer JH, et al. T1G3 bladder cancer—indications for early cystectomy. Int Urol Nephrol 2004;36(1):41–4.

[22] Hasui Y, Osada Y, Kitada S, et al. Significance of invasion to the muscularis mucosae on the progression of superficial bladder cancer. Urology 1994; 43:782–6.

[23] Epstein JI, Amin MB, Reuter V, et al. The World Health Organization/International Society of Urological Pathology classification of urothelial (transitional cell) neoplasms of the urinary bladder. Am J Surg Pathol 1998;22:1435–48.

[24] Cheng L, Weaver AL, Neumann RM, et al. Substaging of T1 bladder carcinoma based on the depth of invasion as measured by micrometer: a new proposal. Cancer 1999;86(6):1035–43.

[25] Platz CE, Cohen MB, Jones MP, et al. Is microstaging of early invasive cancer of the urinary bladder possible or useful?. Mod Pathol 1996;9(11):1035–9.

[26] Epstein JI, Amin MB, Reuter VR, et al. The World Health Organization/International Society of Urological Pathology consensus classification of urothelial (transitional cell) neoplasms of the urinary bladder: Bladder Consensus Conference Committee. Am J Surg Pathol 1998;22(12):1435–48.

[27] Dutta SC, Smith JA Jr, Shappell SB, et al. Clinical under staging of high risk nonmuscle invasive urothelial carcinoma treated with radical cystectomy. J Urol 2001;166(2):490–3.

[28] Wood DP Jr, Montie JE, Pontes JE, et al. Transitional cell carcinoma of the prostate in cystoprostatectomy specimens removed for bladder cancer. J Urol 1989;141(2):346–9.

[29] Amling CL, Thrasher JB, Frazier HA, et al. Radical cystectomy for stages Ta, Tis and T1 transitional cell carcinoma of the bladder. J Urol 1994;151(1):31–5; discussion, 35–6.

[30] Stein JP, Skinner DG. Results with radical cystectomy for treating bladder cancer: a "reference standard" for high-grade, invasive bladder cancer. BJU Int 2003;92(1):12–7.

[31] Pagano F, Bassi P, Galetti TP, et al. Results of contemporary radical cystectomy for invasive bladder cancer: a clinicopathological study with an emphasis on the inadequacy of the tumor, nodes and metastases classification. J Urol 1991;145(1):45–50.

[32] Soloway MS, Lopez AE, Patel J, et al. Results of radical cystectomy for transitional cell carcinoma of the bladder and the effect of chemotherapy. Cancer 1994;73(7):1926–31.

[33] Ghoneim MA, el-Mekresh MM, el-Baz MA, et al. Radical cystectomy for carcinoma of the bladder: critical evaluation of the results in 1026 cases. J Urol 1997;158(2):393–9.

[34] Freeman JA, Esrig D, Stein JP, et al. Radical cystectomy for high risk patients with superficial bladder cancer in the era of orthotopic urinary reconstruction. Cancer 1995;76(5):833–9.

[35] Bianco FJ Jr, Justa D, Grignon DJ, et al. Management of clinical T1 bladder transitional cell carcinoma by radical cystectomy. Urol Oncol 2004; 22(4):290–4.

[36] Paik ML, Scolieri MJ, Brown SL, et al. Limitations of computerized tomography in staging invasive bladder cancer before radical cystectomy. J Urol 2000;163(6):1693–6.

[37] Herr HW. Routine CT scan in cystectomy patients: does it change management? Urology 1996;47(3):324–5.

[38] Miladi M, Peyromaure M, Zerbib M, et al. The value of a second transurethral resection in evaluating patients with bladder tumours. Eur Urol 2003;43(3):241–5.

[39] Herr HW. The value of a second transurethral resection in evaluating patients with bladder tumors. J Urol 1999;162(1):74–6.

[40] Grimm MO, Steinhoff C, Simon X, et al. Effect of routine repeat transurethral resection for superficial bladder cancer: a long-term observational study. J Urol 2003;170(2 Pt 1):433–7.

[41] Rigaud J, Karam G, Braud G, et al. T1 bladder tumors: value of a second endoscopic resection [article in French]. Prog Urol 2002;12(1):27–30.

[42] Herr HW. Neoadjuvant chemotherapy for invasive bladder cancer. Semin Surg Oncol 1989;5(4):266–71.

[43] Cookson MS, Herr HW, Zhang ZF, et al. The treated natural history of high risk superficial bladder cancer: 15-year outcome. J Urol 1997;158(1):62–7.

[44] Joudi FN, O'Donnell MA. Second-line intravesical therapy versus cystectomy for bacille Calmette-Guerin (BCG) failures. Curr Opin Urol 2004;14(5):271–5.

[45] Esrig D, Freeman JA, Stein JP, et al. Early cystectomy for clinical stage T1 transitional cell carcinoma of the bladder. Semin Urol Oncol 1997;15(3):154–60.

[46] Stein JP, Lieskovsky G, Cote R, et al. Radical cystectomy in the treatment of invasive bladder cancer: long-term results in 1054 patients. J Clin Oncol 2001;19(3):666–75.

[47] Stockle M, Alken P, Engelmann U, et al. Radical cystectomy—often too late? Eur Urol 1987;13(6):361–7.

[48] Hautmann RE, Paiss T. Does the option of the ileal neobladder stimulate patient and physician decision toward earlier cystectomy? J Urol 1998;159(6):1845–50.

[49] Cookson MS, Chang SS, Wells N, et al. Complications of radical cystectomy for nonmuscle invasive disease: comparison with muscle invasive disease. J Urol 2003;169(1):101–4.

[50] Stroumbakis N, Herr HW, Cookson MS, et al. Radical cystectomy in the octogenarian. J Urol 1997;158(6):2113–7.

[51] Rosario DJ, Becker M, Anderson JB. The changing pattern of mortality and morbidity from radical cystectomy. BJU Int 2000;85(4):427–30.

[52] Figueroa AJ, Stein JP, Dickinson M, et al. Radical cystectomy for elderly patients with bladder carcinoma: an updated experience with 404 patients. Cancer 1998;83(1):141–7.

[53] Chang SS, Alberts G, Cookson MS, et al. Radical cystectomy is safe in elderly patients at high risk. J Urol 2001;166(3):938–41.

[54] Chang SS, Hassan JM, Cookson MS, et al. Delaying radical cystectomy for muscle invasive bladder cancer results in worse pathological stage. J Urol 2003;170(4 Pt 1):1085–7.

[55] Wallace DM, Bryan RT, Dunn JA, et al. Delay and survival in bladder cancer. BJU Int 2002;89(9):868–78.

[56] Hara I, Miyake H, Hara S, et al. Optimal timing of radical cystectomy for patients with invasive transitional cell carcinoma of the bladder. Jpn J Clin Oncol 2002;32(1):14–8.

[57] Gschwend JE, Vieweg J, Fair WR. Early versus delayed cystectomy for invasive bladder cancer: impact of disease specific survival? J Urol 1997;157:1507a.

[58] Gschwend JE. Outcome of patients undergoing radical cystectomy for invasive bladder cancer. Front Radiat Ther Oncol 2002;36:106–17.

[59] Dalbagni G, Genega E, Hashibe M, et al. Cystectomy for bladder cancer: a contemporary series. J Urol 2001;165(4):1111–6.

[60] Frazier HA, Robertson JE, Dodge RK, et al. The value of pathologic factors in predicting cancer-specific survival among patients treated with radical cystectomy for transitional cell carcinoma of the bladder and prostate. Cancer 1993;71(12):3993–4001.

[61] Stein JP. Indications for early cystectomy. Semin Urol Oncol 2000;18(4):289–95.

ELSEVIER
SAUNDERS

Urol Clin N Am 32 (2005) 157–164

UROLOGIC
CLINICS
of North America

Surgical Factors in the Treatment of Superficial and Invasive Bladder Cancer

Harry W. Herr, MD

Department of Urology, Sidney Kimmel Center for Prostate and Urologic Cancers,
Memorial Sloan-Kettering Cancer Center, 1275 York Avenue, New York, NY 10021, USA

Successful treatment of bladder cancer depends on multiple factors involving both tumor and patient. These include features of the primary tumor (tumor type, stage, and grade); tumor biology (capacity to recur, invade, and metastasize); patient characteristics (general health and quality-of-life concerns); and treatment strategy (selection and type). Surgery remains the predominant treatment of primary, recurrent, and locally advanced bladder tumors, and mounting evidence suggests that surgical factors related to the quality of surgery influence bladder cancer outcomes. Regarding surgery, who performs it and how well it is done for both superficial and invasive bladder cancer matters [1].

Superficial bladder tumors

Bladder tumors are diagnosed by transurethral biopsy and resection. Transurethral resection (TUR) is often regarded as a stochastic procedure that is diagnostic, but only sometimes therapeutic for superficial and minimally invasive bladder tumors. An initial TUR of bladder tumors has three main goals: (1) TUR provides pathologic material to determine the histologic type and grade of bladder tumor; (2) TUR determines the presence, depth, and type of tumor invasion; and (3) TUR aims to remove all visible superficial and invasive tumors. A more complete TUR provides more tissue for pathologic evaluation and results in better staging. Such information is critical because tumor stage, grade, extent, and pattern of growth direct additional therapy and influence

prognosis. A better TUR also provides better local control of superficial tumors.

Prerequisite to successful control of superficial bladder tumors is complete eradication of disease by a thorough TUR done before intravesical therapy. TUR should be wide and deep, especially for papillary or nodular neoplasms suspected of invasion. Proof of this concept is illustrated by a study in which 35% of 462 patients undergoing a TUR had residual tumor in the tumor base and at least 2 cm lateral to visible tumor on wider resection [2]. Studies also show residual tumor at the first follow-up cystoscopy in 41% to 76% of patients [3–5], suggesting that the first resection is often incomplete. Early response to therapy (at 3 or 6 months) after TUR and intravesical therapy of superficial bladder tumors is the most powerful predictor of tumor recurrence and stage progression. Such information combined provides compelling evidence that the quality of the initial TUR is an integral component of treatment determining that first response and subsequent outcome.

How well TURs are performed for bladder tumors varies widely among urologists. For example, the presence of tumor at the first cystoscopy varied from 3% to 46% among a total of 2410 patients with superficial bladder tumors entered in multiple cooperative group trials. There was substantial difference between institutions and surgeons not explained by disease-related factors, suggesting that the quality of the TUR was responsible [6]. Even in the hands of experienced urologists, incomplete resection of minimally invasive bladder tumors is common. Of 71 patients with newly diagnosed stage T1 bladder cancers resected by the author, 18 (25%) had residual T1 disease found on contemporary

E-mail address: herrh@mskcc.org

reresection 4 weeks later and 2 (3%) were up-staged to muscle invasion [7]. Another study showed that 40% of superficially invasive tumors had no muscle submitted or identified in the deep margins of resection [8], and a recent pathology review found that muscularis propria was missing in up to 51% of TUR specimens submitted by general urologists [9]. Proper execution of TUR is critical for primary tumor staging and determining definitive treatment. The pathologist can only evaluate what the urologist submits. Lack of a complete resection significantly increases the chance of understaging, early tumor recurrence, and stage progression of disease.

Second or restaging transurethral resection

Although most urologists agree that ideally initial TUR of bladder tumors should be thorough and complete, many factors confound the adequacy of resection, including multiplicity, size, location, and extent of tumor burden; capability and perseverance of the surgeon; and to some degree the body habitus of the patient. Because local tumor control and accurate tumor staging depend on complete TUR, a second or restaging TUR may be of value in evaluating patients with superficial bladder tumors. The purpose of a restaging TUR is to reduce the uncertainty of depth of tumor invasion, to control the primary tumors better, and to provide additional pathologic information that may help select appropriate treatment.

Table 1 shows results of a second TUR performed by the author in 96 consecutive cases 2 to 6 weeks after initial TUR by multiple referring urologists diagnosed superficial bladder

tumors [8]. A significant proportion (75%) was found on the second TUR to have residual tumor: 31% had noninvasive tumor, 24% had submucosal invasion, and 20% were upstaged to muscle-invasive tumors. An incomplete initial resection was observed in 49% of stage T1 tumors when no muscle was submitted in the TUR specimen compared with 14% when muscle was identified. If cases of carcinoma in situ are excluded because complete TUR is less likely for such tumors, and one considers only the 76 patients with papillary Ta or T1 tumors, then 24% had no residual tumor found on restaging TUR, whereas 76% had residual tumor. Results of the second resection changed the strategy of tumor management in 33% of patients. Table 2 shows results from recently reported series of restaging TUR in patients with stage T1 bladder cancer [10]. Residual T1 tumor was present in 15% to 53% of cases, and another 4% to 29% were upstaged to muscle invasion. Collectively, these data show that a second or restaging TUR improves the quality of TUR, resulting in better assessment, local control, and staging accuracy of superficial bladder tumors.

Can a second TUR improve the treatment outcome of patients presenting with superficial bladder tumors? A recent long-term observational study showed that among a cohort of 124 consecutive patients, a restaging TUR found residual tumor in 33% of cases, and 81% of these were at the original tumor site [11]. After 5 years follow-up, 63% of the patients undergoing a second TUR had tumor-free bladders compared with 40% after a single TUR. Progression to muscle invasion was observed in only two (3%) patients after a restaging TUR. Another recent study suggests that a restaging TUR of high-risk

Table 1
Comparison of bladder tumor stage after first and second transurethral resections

Stage at first TUR	No. pts.	Stage at second TUR. No. pts. (%)			
		T0	Ta/Tis	T1	T2
Tis	20	6 (30)	8 (40)	4 (20)	2 (10)
Ta	18	5 (28)	7 (39)	5 (28)	1 (5)
T1	58	13 (22)	15 (26)	14 (24)	16 (28)
Muscle	35	9 (26)	11 (31)	10 (29)	5 (14)
No muscle	23	4 (17)	4 (17)	4 (17)	11 (49)
Totals	96	72 (75%)			

Abbreviation: TUR, transurethral resection.

Table 2
Bladder tumor stage after second transurethral resection of T1 tumors

Series	Year	No. patients	Stage at 2nd TUR			
			% T0	% Ta/Tis	% T1	% T2
Klan	1991	46		15	26	2
Herr	1999	58	22	26	24	28
Schwaibold	2000	60		17	24	5
Jakse	2001	42	35	17	24	24
Ozen	2001	28		18	53	29
Schips	2002	76	67	11	15	8
Rigaud	2002	52		16	17	4
Vogeli	2003	19		37	43	19

superficial bladder cancers seems to improve the initial response to bacillus Calmette-Guérin therapy [12]. Table 3 shows frequency of tumor recurrence and stage progression among 347 patients with newly diagnosed Ta and T1 bladder tumors according to whether or not they received a restaging TUR before bacillus Calmette-Guérin therapy. Of 132 patients having a single TUR, 75 (57%) had residual tumor at the first follow-up cystoscopy and 45 (34%) later progressed (within 3 years) compared with 62 (29%) of 215 patients who recurred and 16 (7%) who progressed after a restaging TUR. Routine restaging TUR enhances the overall quality of cystoscopic assessment of bladder tumors and becomes more useful as a staging and therapeutic procedure of both Ta and T1 tumors.

TUR of bladder tumors is both diagnostic and therapeutic for non–muscle invasive bladder tumors. A restaging TUR improves staging accuracy and improves local control of superficial and minimally invasive bladder tumors. A second or restaging TUR is recommended for all T1 tumors, multiple high-grade Ta tumors, and in all cases including carcinoma in situ where an initial TUR fails to clear the bladder of visible or suspected tumor. A routine restaging TUR of at least high-risk superficial bladder tumors improves the initial response to intravesical therapy, reduces the frequency of subsequent tumor recurrences, and seems to prevent or delay early tumor progression.

Although TUR of bladder tumors is an essential procedure familiar to urologists, it is difficult to perform well and may not always achieve its desired goals. A complete (or as near complete as possible) TUR identifies characteristics and extent of bladder tumors, providing the best method available to define individual tumor biology. In the present era of molecular medicine, high-technology imaging, and perhaps better drugs, the preliminary TUR has become a forgotten and lost art. An aggressive TUR (and restaging TUR), if it is done well, is one of the most successful and powerful surgical procedures available to the urologist. Indeed, the TUR alone is the most important diagnostic, staging, and therapeutic modality for most bladder tumors. Its success or failure and that of subsequent treatments of superficial bladder tumors depend directly on the ability of the urologist and quality of TUR he or she performs.

Locally advanced bladder cancer

Radical cystectomy with a pelvic lymph node dissection (PLND) is the mainstay treatment of muscle-invasive bladder cancer [13]. The curative intent of radical surgery is to remove all cancer in the bladder, pelvis, and regional lymph nodes. The extent of the primary bladder cancer and the lymph node tumor burden are important prognostic variables in patients undergoing cystectomy. Largely ignored as important factors determining bladder cancer outcome has been the quality of radical cystectomy and the extent of the PLND. The quality of cystectomy depends on several poorly defined factors.

One is the experience of the surgeon. Experienced urologic oncologists operating in high-volume centers tend to achieve better survival results than urologic surgeons who perform few cases in low-volume institutions. Another factor is that many urologists consider it futile to resect locally advanced or node-positive bladder cancers. Higher morbidity and uncertain surgical benefit because of the likelihood of distant metastasis are often cited to justify a lack of surgical aggressiveness for extravesical tumors. A third reason is the

Table 3
Frequency of tumor recurrence and progression by tumor type and restaging TUR

Tumor type (N)	ReTUR (N)	Tumor @ 1st cysto N (%)	Tumor @ 6 mo N (%)	Tumor @ 12 mo N (%)	Progression[a] N (%)
Ta (250)	No (102)	55 (54)	58 (57)	59 (58)	32 (31)
	Yes (148)	46 (31)	35 (24)	24 (16)	11 (7)
T1 (97)	No (30)	20 (67)	22 (73)	21 (70)	13 (43)
	Yes (67)	16 (24)	14 (21)	12 (18)	5 (8)
All (347)	No (132)	75 (57)	80 (61)	80 (61)	45 (34)
	Yes (215)	62 (29)	49 (23)	36 (17)	16 (7)

Abbreviations: N, number of patients; TUR, transurethral resection.
[a] Stage progression (Ta to $=/>$ T1, T1 to $=/>$ T2) within 3 years. P $= .001$ for all differences between one or two TURs.

age and health of the patient. Surgeons may perform a less radical operation in aged or infirm patients, to reduce operating time and lessen morbidity associated with longer and more extensive surgery. Surgery also aims to identify patients who are likely to develop recurrent disease and candidates for chemotherapy. Both cure and accurate staging depend on the quality of surgery. For example, earlier literature suggested that survival after cystectomy in patients with positive nodes was only 7% to 15%, but more recent series have shown that survival is now up to 35% [13]. Although some of this change can be ascribed to stage migration, there is evidence that surgical technique is also a predictive factor.

Radical cystectomy is defined as the wide resection of all perivesical fat and tissue around the bladder and adjacent organs, to achieve a negative surgical margin. The plane of dissection is the musculoskeletal boundaries of the pelvis. A standard PLND removes all of the distal common iliac, external iliac, obturator, and hypogastric nodes. Such dissection yields an average of 10 to 14 nodes. An extended lymph node dissection to the aortic bifurcation including the presacral nodes often yields 20 to 40 nodes. How often is radical cystectomy done with a complete pelvic node dissection, and does it matter?

The author has shown that a thorough PLND increasing the number of lymph nodes removed influences bladder cancer outcomes [14]. Fig. 1 and Table 4 show survival after radical cystectomy and pelvic lymphadenectomy in 637 patients stratified by node-examined quartiles [15]. For

Table 4
Outcome by number of nodes examined (quartiles) in 637 patients

No. of nodes	No. pts.	% Local recurrence rate	% 10-year survival rate
0–5	149	26	33
6–10	152	13	49
11–14	157	9	73
>14	179	5	79

both node-negative and node-positive patients, improved survival and reduced local recurrence rates were associated with greater number of lymph nodes removed. Presumably, fewer nodes removed risks leaving microscopic positive nodes in the pelvis, contributing to later relapse and reduced overall survival.

Others have also provided convincing arguments that extending the limits of lymph node dissection (and removing more nodes) beyond the standard pelvic node dissection may confer additional therapeutic benefit in both node-negative [16] and node-positive patients [17,18]. The author has found in a prospective evaluation of 144 patients undergoing radical cystectomy that among patients with unexpected microscopic positive nodes, 33% involved the common iliac nodes [19], suggesting that the node dissection must at least extend above the true pelvis to be reasonably sure that all regional metastatic disease is resected. The author also demonstrated that by submitting nodes as separate nodal packets, node counts varied only with the extent of

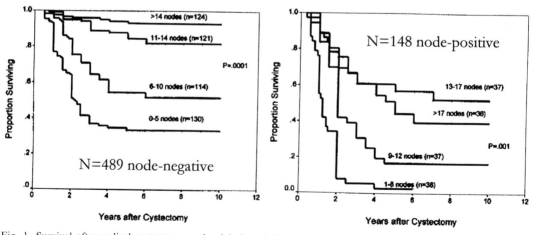

Fig. 1. Survival after radical cystectomy and pelvic lymphadenectomy in 637 patients stratified by node-examined quartiles.

node dissection and not pathologic evaluation. Separate submission of resected nodal tissue according to defined templates of dissection assists the pathologist to identify presence or absence of regional disease and to provide feedback to the surgeon regarding the quality of his or her cystectomy and pelvic node dissection.

Despite compelling evidence that quality of cystectomy matters, the problem with retrospective studies is that they are from single academic institutions where surgery was performed by a limited number of surgeons. The author attempted to overcome this objection by evaluating measures of surgical quality using data from the recently reported randomized cooperative group trial (SWOG 8710, INT-0080) comparing neoadjuvant chemotherapy plus cystectomy with cystectomy alone for locally advanced bladder cancer [20]. In 268 patients who underwent cystectomy by 106 surgeons in 109 different institutions, the author evaluated the influence of surgical factors on overall survival and local recurrence [21]. These factors included surgical margin status, extent of node dissection as evidenced by type of dissection and number of lymph nodes examined, whether the surgeon was a general urologist or a specialist trained in urologic oncology, and whether surgery was done at an academic or community center.

First, the author found that surgical factors were not altered by chemotherapy, which is not surprising because this comparative study showed a survival advantage for neoadjuvant chemotherapy. More importantly, with multivariate modeling adjusting for well-known risk factors influencing survival or local recurrence, such as pathologic stage and age, the most important negative factors were whether the surgical margins were positive and whether fewer than 10 lymph nodes were removed. Fig. 2 shows that the number of nodes removed influenced survival even if the nodes were negative for cancer. Fig. 3 shows that a standard pelvic node dissection to the bifurcation of the common iliac vessels was associated with significantly longer survival times than a dissection limited only to the obturator space or no dissection at all. Fig. 4 shows that neoadjuvant chemotherapy improved survival only in patients who had a high-quality cystectomy and pelvic node dissection. A more extended pelvic node dissection removing more nodes reduced the positive margin rate, provided a better wide-margin resection of the bladder, and contributed to better survival regardless of whether or not patients received neoadjuvant chemotherapy.

Patients who underwent radical cystectomy and standard template PLND achieved a negative surgical margin and had more lymph nodes removed, and had superior postcystectomy survival than patients who had less favorable surgical features. A positive surgical margin, regardless of node status or total number of nodes removed, was associated with a local recurrence and death as a result of bladder cancer. The 5-year survival rate for patients having cystectomy and no, limited, or standard lymph node dissection was 33%, 46%, and 60%, respectively. The 5-year survival rate for patients with fewer than 10 nodes removed was 44% compared with 61% for patients with more than 10 nodes examined. Local recurrences occurred in only 6% of patients after radical cystectomy and standard pelvic node

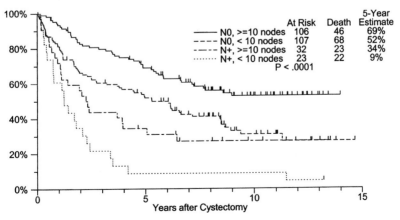

Fig. 2. Postcystectomy survival by node status and number of nodes removed.

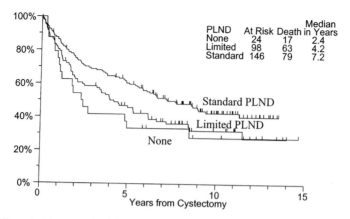

Fig. 3. Overall survival by type of pelvic lymph node dissection. PLND, pelvic lymph node dissection.

dissection removing more than 10 nodes, compared with 25% after a limited node dissection with fewer than 10 nodes. Half the patients who had no node dissection had a local recurrence. The importance of locoregional control is emphasized by the fact that 91% of the 41 patients (15%) who had a local recurrence died as a result of bladder cancer, including all 25 patients who had positive surgical margins. The fact that both surgical margins and number of nodes were independent predictors of postcystectomy survival and local recurrence in multivariate models suggests that the quality of surgery significantly influences bladder cancer outcomes.

The author then extended the inquiry to discover whether these surgical quality factors were related to the type of surgeon and institution. It was found that surgeons specifically trained in urologic oncology were more likely to achieve

negative margins, perform at least a standard PLND, and remove more than 10 nodes than were general urologists. Although there were many exceptions, patients operated on by urologic oncologists, largely in academic centers, enjoyed better survival and fewer local recurrences than those operated on by community urologists.

The data show that reduced local recurrence and better survival were associated with negative surgical margins and higher node counts (as surrogate marker for the extent of PLND). These two significant surgical variables are interrelated and depend on the experience of the surgeon and thoroughness of the pelvic node dissection. The author demonstrated substantial variability in the type of surgical resection and hence the number of lymph nodes removed. Quality of radical cystectomy is critical to local control and survival of locally advanced bladder cancer. This conclusion

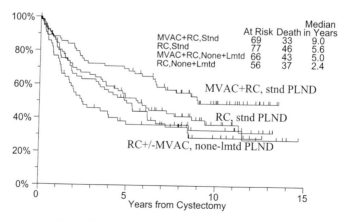

Fig. 4. Survival by treatment and type of pelvic lymph node dissection for Southwest Oncology Group 8710 patients receiving cystectomy. Lmtd, limited; MVAC, methotrexate, vinblastine, Adriamycin, cisplatin; RC, radical cystectomy; Stnd, standard.

is especially compelling because it is derived from a multicenter study involving many surgeons and institutions rather than from a single surgeon or center experience.

The need to secure and retain local and regional control of invasive bladder cancers, even extravesical tumors with positive nodes, will assume increasing importance as systemic therapy improves and reduces deaths from distant metastases. Accepted surgical standards for radical cystectomy and PLND should be established and validated prospectively. Given that node counts are related to both margins and outcome, a minimum number should be agreed on as a proxy measure of the quality of surgery. This is important not only for individual patient management but also for the design and evaluation of combined modality studies in bladder cancer. Improving the general quality of surgery may even prove to be as or more important than anticipated improvements in chemotherapy regimens.

Summary

Tumor stage, grade, and variations in biologic behavior are primary features that largely determine bladder cancer outcomes. Quality of surgery used to assess and treat bladder tumors is critical to a successful outcome. Diagnosis, prognosis, local tumor control, and survival are highly dependent on surgical factors associated with the quality of surgical methods. In cases of superficial bladder tumors, this involves an aggressive TUR of all visible and suspected tumors, including a second resection in most cases. For invasive bladder cancers, radical cystectomy and a complete PLND are required. Both procedures require a high level of skill to achieve a successful outcome. Urologists have no control over the extent of disease or tumor biology, but can control how they evaluate and treat patients. The challenge is how to get better at maximizing surgical efforts. The who and how of surgery in bladder cancer does indeed matter.

References

[1] Lange PH, Lin DW. Does the who and how of surgery in bladder cancer matter? J Clin Oncol 2004;22:2762.

[2] Kolozsy Z. Histopathological "self-control" in TUR of bladder tumors. Br J Urol 1991;67:162.

[3] Solsona E, Iborra I, Dumont R, et al. The 3-month clinical response to intravesical therapy as a predictive factor for progression in patients with superficial bladder cancer. J Urol 2000;164:685.

[4] Holmang S, Johannson SL. Stage Ta-T1 bladder cancer: the relationship between finding at first cystoscopy and subsequent tumor recurrence and progression. J Urol 2002;167:1634–7.

[5] Andius P, Holmang S. BCG therapy in stage Ta/T1 bladder cancer: prognostic factors for time to recurrence and progression. BJU Int 2004;93:980.

[6] Brausi M, Collette L, Kurth K, et al. Variability in the recurrence rate at first follow-up cystoscopy after TUR in TaT1 transitional cell carcinoma of the bladder: a combined analysis of seven EORTC studies. Eur Urol 2002;41:523.

[7] Dalbagni G, Herr HW, Reuter VE. Impact of a second transurethral resection on the staging of T1 bladder cancer. Urology 2002;60:822.

[8] Herr HW. The value of a second transurethral resection in evaluating patients with bladder tumors. J Urol 1999;162:74.

[9] Maruniak NA, Takezawa K, Murphy WM. Accurate pathological staging of urothelial neoplasms requires better cystoscopic sampling. J Urol 2002;167:2404.

[10] Herr HW. Transurethral resection of bladder tumors. In: Schoenberg M, editor. Current management of bladder tumors. 2005, In press.

[11] Grimm MC, Ackermann R, Vogeli TA. Effect of routine repeat transurethral resection for superficial bladder cancer: a long-term observational study. J Urol 2003;170:433.

[12] Herr HW. A restaging TUR of high-risk superficial bladder cancers improves the initial response to BCG therapy. J Urol, in press.

[13] Stein JP, Lieskovsky G, Cote R, et al. Radical cystectomy in the treatment of invasive bladder cancer: long-term results in 1,054 patients. J Clin Oncol 2001;19:666.

[14] Herr HW, Bochner BH, Dalbagni G, et al. Impact of the number of lymph nodes retrieved on outcome in patients with muscle invasive bladder cancer. J Urol 2002;167:1295.

[15] Herr HW. Extent of surgery and pathology evaluation has an impact on bladder cancer outcomes after radical cystectomy. Urology 2003;61:105.

[16] Poulson AL, Horn T, Steven K. Radical cystectomy; extending limits of pelvic lymph node dissection improves survival for patients with bladder cancer confined to the bladder wall. J Urol 1998;160:2015.

[17] Leissner J, Ghoneim MA, Abol-Enein H, et al. Extended lymphadenectomy in patients with urothelial bladder cancer: results of prospective multicenter study. J Urol 2004;171:139.

[18] Stein JP, Skinner DG. Results with radical cystectomy for treating bladder cancer: a "reference standard" for high-grade, invasive bladder cancer. BJU Int 2003;92:12.

[19] Bochner BH, Cho D, Herr HW, et al. Prospectively packaged lymph node dissections with radical cystectomy: evaluation of node variability and node mapping. J Urol 2004;172:1286.

[20] Grossman HB, Natale RB, Tangen CM, et al. Neoadjuvant chemotherapy plus cystectomy compared with cystectomy alone for locally advanced bladder cancer. N Engl J Med 2003;349:859.

[21] Herr HW, Faulkner JR, Grossman HB, et al. Surgical factors influence bladder cancer outcomes: a cooperative group report. J Clin Oncol 2004;22: 2781.

ELSEVIER
SAUNDERS

Urol Clin N Am 32 (2005) 165–175

UROLOGIC
CLINICS
of North America

Clinical Indications and Outcomes with Nerve-sparing Cystectomy in Patients with Bladder Cancer

Thomas M. Kessler, MD, Fiona C. Burkhard, MD, Urs E. Studer, MD*

Department of Urology, University of Bern, CH-3010 Bern, Switzerland

Until recently, evaluation of outcome after radical cystectomy was based mainly on oncologic results. However, with constantly improving survival of these patients the question of the impact of radical cystectomy and urinary diversion on quality of life has emerged. Preserved sexual function and, in the case of an orthotopic bladder substitute, an intact body image and normal voiding function based on an adequate neobladder capacity and complete urinary continence allow patients to achieve a normal life style. The role of nerve-sparing surgery to attain these goals is a matter of intense debate. It has been shown that nerve sparing does have a positive impact on erectile function and urinary continence after ileal orthotopic bladder substitution [1,2]. On the other hand, some concern has arisen regarding radical tumor resection if nerve sparing is attempted. However, studies exist demonstrating that oncologic outcome is not compromised by a nerve-sparing technique in carefully selected patients and, in particular, the rate of local recurrences is not increased [3–5]. Based on these considerations we believe that nerve sparing should be attempted if possible. In this article, patient selection criteria, aspects of surgical technique, and the current literature are discussed.

Anatomic and physiologic considerations

Autonomic innervation of the pelvic organs

The autonomic nervous system supplies the lower urinary tract with afferent and efferent nerve fibers. The sympathetic nerve fibers originate from the intermediolateral gray matter of the spinal cord segments T10–L2 and pass through the ventral root into the white ramus communicans and then to the sympathetic trunk. From there on they proceed via the lumbar splanchnic nerves, at first lateral to, and then in front of, the aorta (on the right side para-/retrocavally) into the intermesenteric plexus and on to the superior hypogastric plexus at the level of the aortic bifurcation. The superior hypogastric plexus splits into the left and right hypogastric nerves that pass inferolaterally along the perirectal fascia medial to the ureter and just beneath the peritoneum on both sides toward the pelvic plexus (inferior hypogastric plexus). This is situated anterolaterally to the sigmoidorectal junction. Parasympathetic nerve fibers arising from the intermediolateral cell column of the sacral cord S2–S4 run in the pelvic splanchnic nerves along the lateral aspect of the rectum to join the hypogastric nerves and form the pelvic plexus. The pelvic plexus consists of a variable network of both sympathetic and parasympathetic fibers and is located lateral to the rectum, bladder, seminal vesicles, and prostate/vagina (Figs. 1 and 2). Additional fibers join the pelvic plexus directly from the sacral sympathetic ganglia. Mixed sympathetic and parasympathetic fibers pass from the pelvic plexus to supply the pelvic viscera with a dual autonomic innervation. Autonomic fibers from the pelvic plexus, including afferent and efferent fibers, innervate the rectum and the urogenital tract and end as the paraprostatic neurovascular bundle or paravaginal plexus before supplying the urogenital diaphragm, sphincter, and erectile organs.

* Corresponding author.
 E-mail address: urs.studer@insel.ch (U.E. Studer).

0094-0143/05/$ - see front matter © 2005 Elsevier Inc. All rights reserved.
doi:10.1016/j.ucl.2005.02.005

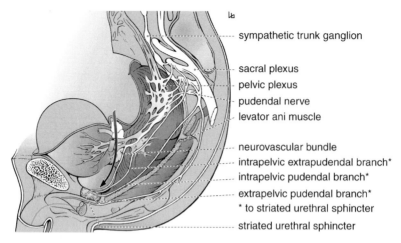

Fig. 1. Innervation of the pelvic organs in the male. The *arrow* indicates the line of dissection on the non–tumor-bearing side when performing nerve-sparing cystectomy.

Sphincter innervation

Although the neuroanatomy and physiology of the urinary continence mechanism is not yet completely understood, there is evidence that both the somatic pudendal nerve and autonomic branches of the pelvic plexus are involved in the male [6] and female [7]. Somatic motor innervation passes from Onuf's nucleus in the anterior horn of the sacral segments S2–S4 and travels to the external urethral sphincter via an intra- and an extrapelvic branch of the pudendal nerve. Additional intrapelvic extrapudendal nerve fibers from S2–S3 initially pass just lateral to the pelvic plexus

and then along the dorsolateral surface of the rectum until they disappear into the levator ani muscle and terminate in the external urethral sphincter [8]. However, autonomic fibers also play a role in urethral sphincter innervation.

In the male, sympathetic stimulation results in bladder neck closure by smooth muscle contraction, thus contributing to urinary continence and preventing reflux of ejaculate into the bladder. The importance of an intact bladder neck is shown by its ability to maintain urinary continence even when the external urethral sphincter has been damaged by traumatic pudendal nerve injury or neurologic diseases. On the other hand,

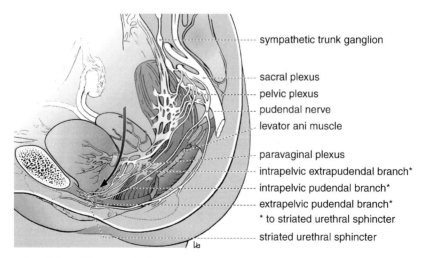

Fig. 2. Innervation of the pelvic organs in the female. The *arrow* indicates the line of dissection on the non–tumor-bearing side when performing nerve-sparing cystectomy.

in patients with a completely incompetent bladder neck due to bladder neck incision or transurethral resection, urinary continence is maintained by an intact external urethral sphincter. The effect of the autonomic innervation on the sphincteric mechanism could be convincingly shown by intraoperative stimulation of the neurovascular bundle during radical retropubic prostatectomy. This results in significant increases in urethral pressure [9]. In addition to the efferent autonomic and somatic nerve fibers innervating the sphincteric musculature, intrapelvic afferents from the membranous urethra contribute to urinary continence [10]. Intact proximal sensation leads to improved urinary continence due to a conscious or unconscious sensation of urine entering the membranous urethra. This induces either a spinal reflex or a voluntary sphincter contraction resulting in an increased tone of the external urethral sphincter and pelvic floor. These afferent nerve fibers from the membranous urethra are postulated to run in branches of the pelvic plexus or the intrapelvic pudendal nerve, which are prone to iatrogenic damage during radical pelvic surgery.

In the female, the bladder neck (proximal urethra) is a far weaker structure than in the male, but incompetence also predisposes to urinary incontinence. Thus, urinary incontinence following radical hysterectomy seems mainly due to iatrogenic autonomic nerve damage. Indeed, decreased maximum urethral closure pressure and shortened functional urethral length was reported after Wertheim's hysterectomy [11]. Further support comes from animal studies showing that stimulation of the pelvic nerves following a nerve-sparing cystectomy leads to an increase [12] and autonomic denervation to a decrease in proximal urethral pressure [13]. Moreover, we found similar results in a female patient after non–nerve-sparing radical cystectomy and orthotopic bladder substitution where the proximal third of the urethra lost all of its resting tone and the midurethra about 30% [14]. This supports the view that there are three different innervation patterns in the female urethra. The proximal third is supplied primarily by the autonomic nerves, while the distal third is innervated mainly by the somatic pudendal nerve. The midurethra has equal innervation by both autonomic and somatic nerves.

In the majority of patients somatic innervation by the pudendal nerve alone may be sufficient to maintain sphincteric function. This could explain why some patients remain continent after orthotopic bladder substitution despite non–nerve-sparing surgery. Another reason may be that the nerves are at least partially preserved during cystectomy even when the surgeon had not intended to perform a nerve-sparing procedure. This is especially so because a bilateral resection of the vesical pedicles along the pararectal/presacral plane (which would result in damage of the pelvic plexus) is not always done.

Sexual function

The sympathetic and parasympathetic nervous system both play an important role in sexual function. Sacral parasympathetic fibers from S2–S4 traveling through the pelvic plexus and forming the nervi erigentes dorsolateral to the bladder and prostate are responsible for the blood flow into the corpora cavernosa resulting in penile erection. Sympathetic fibers are responsible for emission of semen from the seminal vesicles into the prostatic urethra and antegrade ejaculation. Thus, iatrogenic damage of the parasympathetic and sympathetic pathways during radical pelvic surgery may result in erectile and ejaculation dysfunction.

In women, parasympathetic activation mediates the release of vasoactive intestinal polypeptide from nerve endings in the vagina. This results in a marked increase in vaginal transudation of fluid which, together with Bartholin's gland secretion, provides adequate vaginal lubrication [15]. In addition, parasympathetic stimulation causes vascular engorgement of the clitoris and labia, analogous to the situation in men. Therefore, parasympathetic nerve lesions most likely result in insufficient lubrication causing vaginal dryness and dyspareunia.

Afferent fibers from the dorsal nerve of the penis/clitoris pass via the pudendal nerve to the sacral spinal cord, which coordinates the sexual response in both women and men. Descending input arrives from higher centers and efferent fibers travel in the sympathetic, parasympathetic, and pudendal nerves.

Bowel function

The autonomic innervation of the rectum is also supplied by fibers from the pelvic plexus so that damage during radical urologic pelvic surgery may result in defecation disorders. Indeed, it has been shown in a recent study [16] that patients undergoing radical prostatectomy do report some degree of postoperative impairment in bowel function. This was short-lived, and bowel function improved significantly during the first 3 months after surgery. In addition, bowel function and bowel bother scores were found to be lower in patients with non–nerve-sparing compared with nerve-sparing radical retropubic prostatectomy [17]. However, the differences were not statistically significant, and it should be taken into consideration that the questionnaires were completed at least 1 year following surgery. Nevertheless, bowel function after radical urologic pelvic surgery is a sparsely investigated issue, and data following radical cystectomy are lacking.

Potential impact of extended lymphadenectomy on nerve sparing

Meticulous pelvic lymphadenectomy may improve the chance of cure in patients with only a few microscopic metastases in normal looking nodes [18]. In addition, meticulous removal of all lymphatic and connective tissue along the external and internal iliac vessels, the obturator fossa, and side wall of the bladder alleviates visualization during cystectomy, and blood transfusions are required in less than 50% of patients [19]. This does not impair nerve sparing surgery as the lymphatic tissue lies lateral to the nerves. If a more extensive resection is attempted (ie, medial to the ureters at the level of the common iliac bifurcation, at the aortic bifurcation or on the interaortic/paraaortic left side), care must be taken to avoid damaging sympathetic nerve fibers descending along the aorta and common iliac bifurcation. Damage to these nerve fibers may have a negative impact on continence and sexual function. The obturator and external/internal iliac lymph nodes represent the primary sentinel lymphatic drainage for bladder cancer [20]. Patients with positive nodes in the paraaortic region generally have additional nodes involved. For this reason, the potential additional benefit of an extended more proximal lymphadenectomy up to the aorta should be carefully weighed against the increased morbidity.

Which patients are suitable for nerve-sparing cystectomy?

Based on the above considerations, sparing of the autonomic innervation (both sympathetic and parasympathetic) is important for preservation of sexual, lower urinary tract, and bowel function. Therefore, we believe that nerve-sparing cystectomy should always be attempted if radical tumor resection is not compromised. Nerve sparing is not only attempted in patients undergoing ileal orthotopic bladder substitution. Also, patients with other forms of urinary diversion with intact sexual function preoperatively may profit from nerve sparing.

- Unilateral nerve sparing is attempted on the non–tumor-bearing side in patients with unilateral tumors. On the tumor-bearing side, no nerve sparing is attempted as the dorsomedial pedicle of the bladder is resected along the pararectal/presacral plane to remove the lymphatics draining the bladder base.
- Bilateral nerve sparing is attempted in patients with tumors located at the bladder dome, the anterior bladder wall, or in patients with multifocal T1 G3 bladder cancer with or without carcinoma in situ.

Tipps and tricks to help minimize nerve damage during cystectomy and orthotopic bladder substitution

For nerve-sparing cystectomy in the male, the nerve fibers in the dorsomedial pedicles lateral to the seminal vesicles as well as the paraprostatic neurovascular bundle have to be spared (Fig. 1). The pelvic plexus can be preserved by sectioning the dorsomedial pedicle along its ventral aspect, anterolateral to the seminal vesicles, and terminating the dissection at the base of the prostate. Care should be taken to avoid even minimal trauma to the pelvic plexus through clamping or pinching of the tissue located on the dorsolateral aspect of the seminal vesicles. After that, a nerve-sparing prostatectomy must be performed. For optimal visualization of the neurovascular bundles and to avoid damage to the autonomic nerves running into the membranous urethra, a lateral approach with incision of the endopelvic and periprostatic fascia and bunching of Santorini's plexus at the level of the prostate and not distal to it is of utmost importance. The dorsolateral neurovascular bundle can be separated from the prostatic capsule (Fig. 3) or the prostatic capsule can be left in place. The prostatic apex is approached laterally directly along the prostatic capsule, and the membranous urethra is delivered sharply out of the donut-shaped prostatic apex to avoid nerve damage on the dorsolateral side of the urethra and to maintain maximum urethral

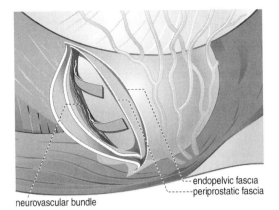

Fig. 3. Following incision of the endopelvic and periprostatic fascia the dorsolateral neurovascular bundle is separated completely from the prostatic capsule.

length. If additional hemostasis of Santorini's plexus is required, one suture is placed in the coronal plane between the venous plexus and the urethra, and then perpendicularly toward the symphysis pubis. This encompasses all the veins and avoids injury of the external sphincter.

For nerve sparing in the female, dissection is performed along the anterolateral paravaginal plane, no further dorsal than the 2 or 10 o'clock position, in an attempt to preserve the paravaginal fibers passing to the urethra (Figs. 2 and 4). An empty sponge-holding forceps in the vagina helps facilitate dissection along the whitish vaginal wall. The vaginal wall is then opened at the level of the cervix and the portion of the anterior vaginal wall adjacent to the trigone is resected en bloc with the bladder 1 cm above the bladder neck. The endopelvic fascia is disturbed as little as possible to minimize damage to the intrapelvic branch of the pudendal nerve, which also contributes to urethral innervation.

To prevent thermal damage to the nerves during cystectomy electrocautery should not be used along the spared neurovascular bundles. If it is necessary to control bleeding from the neurovascular bundle, superficial 4-0 polyglycolic acid sutures are placed and tied loosely. Any trauma caused by squeezing, pulling, or tearing of the pelvic plexus and neurovascular bundles must be avoided.

After construction of the ileal orthotopic bladder substitute particular care should be taken in placing the sutures for the urethro-ileal anastomosis [21]. Two dorsal sutures are passed medial to the neurovascular bundles to avoid damage to the nerves through the remnant of

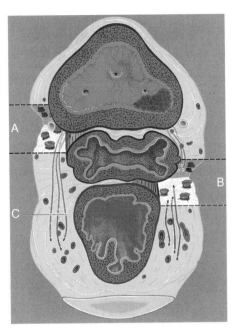

Fig. 4. In women, the dissection extends no further than the 2 or 10 o'clock position on the non–tumor-bearing side (A) preserving the autonomic nerves (C), and extends as far as the pararectal region on the tumor-bearing side (B).

Denonvillier's fascia and the urethral stump (Fig. 5). Two stitches are placed both lateral and ventral to the nerves. The two ventral stitches include only a slight portion of the sphincter muscle and are then placed through the ligated Santorini's plexus to ensure sufficient fixation and avoid traction on the sphincter muscle by the bladder substitute. All sutures are tied loosely to prevent ischemia resulting in stricture and shortening of the functional urethral length.

Outcomes after nerve-sparing radical cystectomy

Oncologic outcome

The aim of radical cystectomy with subsequent urinary diversion is local control of cancer combined with the best possible quality of life. To minimize the risk of compromising radical tumor resection, nerve sparing is only attempted on the non–tumor-bearing side. This requires precise preoperative tumor localization.

In the Johns Hopkins series [3,4] the local recurrence rate following nerve-sparing radical cystectomy was 5%. Following nerve and prostate sparing cystectomy and ileal orthotopic bladder

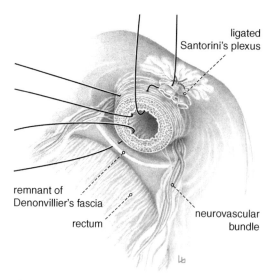

ligated
Santorini's plexus

remnant of
Denonvillier's fascia

rectum

neurovascular
bundle

Fig. 5. For construction of the anastomosis with the ileal orthotopic bladder substitute dorsal sutures are placed through the remnant of Denovillier's fascia and the urethral stump medial to the neurovascular bundles to avoid damage and ventral through the ligated Santorini's plexus to avoid traction on the sphincter muscle.

substitution, Vallancien et al [5] reported local recurrences in 5% of patients with organ-confined tumors (≤pT2, pN0) and 9% of patients with non–organ-confined tumors (>pT2, pN0). In our population, when nerve sparing was possible and attempted (as defined earlier), isolated local recurrences were observed in 3% of patients with organ-confined tumors (≤pT2, pN0), 11% with non–organ-confined tumors (>pT2, pN0), and 13% with positive lymph nodes (any pT, pN+) [22]. Although a direct comparison is not possible due to inherent differences in the patient population, risk factors, selection criteria, and pathologic stage, our results of nerve sparing are comparable to the results of other centers where no special attention was paid to nerve sparing. Stein et al [23] reported a local recurrence rate of 6% and 13% in patients with organ-confined and extravesical lymph node-negative tumors, respectively. Patients with lymph node-positive disease had a 13% local recurrence rate. Hautmann et al reported an overall 12% local recurrence rate following radical cystectomy and ileal orthotopic bladder substitution. Thus, nerve sparing does not appear to compromise cancer control, provided the patients are carefully selected according to tumor localization and extension.

Urinary continence after orthotopic urinary diversion

There are only a few large series assessing the impact of nerve sparing surgery on urinary continence following radical cystectomy and orthotopic bladder substitution in the male [1,2,5]. Daytime and nighttime continence rates, independent of nerve sparing surgery, range from 87% to 98% and 72% to 95%, respectively [2,5,24–26]. When assessing these results it should be taken into account that in a large number of patients the nerves are probably at least partially preserved without the surgeon having attempted a nerve sparing procedure. In addition, direct comparison of the various series is difficult due to differences in the patient populations, risk factors, selection criteria, length of follow-up, definition of continence, and statistical methods. In a recent study, we used multivariate analysis to independently assess factors influencing urinary continence after radical cystoprostatectomy and ileal orthotopic bladder substitution (Table 1). Daytime continence was best and was achieved earlier in patients with preservation of one or both neurovascular bundles than in those without nerve sparing (Fig. 6). This seems to be due to preservation of branches from the pelvic plexus as well as the intrapelvic branch of the pudendal nerve. However, the afferents from the membranous urethra, most likely in branches of the pelvic plexus or the intrapelvic pudendal nerve, also have a positive impact on urinary continence [10].

In women, the role of nerve sparing on voiding function following orthotopic bladder substitution is of intense debate. In our small series using a nerve-sparing technique we observed a daytime and nighttime continence of 100% and 89%, respectively assessed by questionnaire after a median follow-up of 19 months [27]. Excellent results were also reported in other series where no special attention was paid to nerve sparing [28,29]. However, Stenzl et al [30] reported a considerably higher catheterization rate of 72% without nerve sparing compared with 0% to 9% when preservation of the nerves was attempted (Table 2).

In fact, nerve sparing may be more important in women because there is a larger smooth muscle component in the female urethra than in the male membranous urethra [31]. Our present understanding of female urethral function would suggest that optimal continence in female patients is obtained with preservation of a maximum of functional length, that is, with preserved innervation of the

Table 1
Multivariate analysis with urinary continence and recovery of erectile function as outcome variables after radical cystoprostatectomy and ileal orthotopic bladder substitution

	HR	95% CI	P
Daytime continence			
Attempted (uni- or bilateral) nerve sparing versus no attempted nerve sparing	1.4	1.05–1.87	0.023
Nighttime continence			
≤65 years old versus >65 years old	1.39	1.07–1.8	0.014
Recovery of erectile function (reduced or normal erections)			
Attempted (uni- or bilateral) nerve sparing versus no attempted nerve sparing	2.59	1.24–5.39	0.011
≤65 years old versus >65 years old	2.98	1.83–4.85	<0.0001

Abbreviations: HR, hazard ratio; 95% CI, 95% confidence interval for hazard ratio.

    The rate of daytime continence was significantly higher in patients with attempted nerve sparing and nighttime continence was significantly better in patients ≤65 years. Erectile function recovered significantly more often in patients with attempted nerve sparing and in those ≤65 years. (*From* Kessler TM, Burkhard FC, Perimenis P, et al. Attempted nerve sparing surgery and age have a significant effect on urinary continence and erectile function after radical cystoprostatectomy and ileal orthotopic bladder substitution. J Urol 2004;172:1323–7.)

entire urethra. If, however, the autonomic nerves cannot be preserved, a denervated proximal urethra may lead to kinking and outlet obstruction requiring self-catheterization. In these women, resection of the proximal third of the urethra would more likely ensure spontaneous voiding, albeit at the possible price of drop-wise urinary incontinence when walking due to the shortened functional length of the urethra. Typically, these women are not incontinent during the classical stress tests such as coughing, straining, or sneezing, because the spinal reflex to the urethra and pelvic floor by the extrapelvic branch of the pudendal nerve remains intact. However, they may have

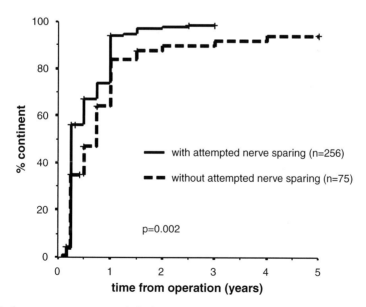

Fig. 6. After radical cystoprostatectomy and ileal orthotopic bladder substitution, attempted nerve sparing was significantly associated with better daytime continence. However, it should be considered that when applying the Kaplan-Meier method patients reporting complete urinary continence from then on remain classified as continent even if they become incontinent later on. (*From* Kessler TM, Burkhard FC, Perimenis P, et al. Attempted nerve sparing surgery and age have a significant effect on urinary continence and erectile function after radical cystoprostatectomy and ileal orthotopic bladder substitution. J Urol 2004;172:1323–7; with permission.)

Table 2
Association between no, uni-, or bilateral nerve-sparing cystectomy with orthotopic bladder substitution and subsequent voiding patterns in 101 women

Nerve sparing	Normal voiding	Obstructive voiding	Clean intermittent catheterization
Bilateral	77% (51/66)	14% (9/66)	9% (6/66)
Unilateral	86% (24/28)	14% (4/28)	0% (0/28)
No	14% (1/7)	14% (1/7)	72% (5/7)

One woman with a permanent catheter after failed bladder neck suspension was not included. (*From* Stenzl A, Jarolim L, Coloby P, et al. Urethra-sparing cystectomy and orthotopic urinary diversion in women with malignant pelvic tumors. Cancer 2001;92:1864–71; with permission.)

leakage when walking, due to a shortened functional urethral length or diminished urethral sensory threshold.

Despite attempted nerve sparing and meticulous attention being paid to preservation of the sphincteric mechanism, good functional results can only be achieved if other factors affecting urinary continence are taken into account. Age-related mechanisms including decreased sphincter length and decreased maximum urethral closure pressure [32] as well as affected urethral innervation in analogy to diminished detrusor innervation [33] may play a role. Indeed, younger age has a positive effect on urinary continence, and remained the only statistically significant factor associated with nighttime continence in our multivariate analysis (Table 2).

In addition, continence after orthotopic bladder substitution is determined by specific characteristics of the reservoir and the outlet mechanism [34–36]. The reservoir should be detubularized and compliant, with a low end-filling pressure, which is influenced by reservoir size. According to Laplace's law, the intraluminal pressure is lower in larger reservoirs with similar tension in the reservoir wall. However, the reservoir should not be too large, as this can result in development of a "floppy bag" and inefficient emptying. Significant postvoid residuals cause infection leading to reservoir overactivity with incontinence and increased mucus production, which in turn, supports urinary tract infection. Furthermore, the absence of neurofeedback to the brain may result in excess capacity and increased intrareservoir pressure, which ultimately exceeds urethral closure pressure and leads to overflow incontinence.

Sexual function

The effect of nerve-sparing radical cystoprostatectomy on sexual function is a sparsely investigated issue. The recovery rate of erectile function ranges from 33% to 100% (Table 3) using a nerve-sparing technique with or without sparing of the prostate. However, similar to the results of urinary continence, direct comparison of the studies is of questionable value because of differences in the patient populations, risk factors, pathologic stage, selection criteria, length of follow-up, definition of sexual/erectile recovery, medical aids, and statistical methods. Thus, various factors may confound the effect of nerve-sparing surgery. For independent evaluation of factors influencing erectile function we applied multivariate analysis and found that a nerve-

Table 3
Reported recovery of erectile/sexual function after nerve-sparing cystectomy

Authors	Erectile/sexual function recovery	Nerve sparing	Time point of evaluation
Schoenberg, Brendler et al, 1996 [4]	42% (33/78)	yes	≥ 1 year
Vallancien et al, 2002 [5]	82% (50/61)	yes[a]	1 year
Meinhardt and Horenblas, 2003 [39]	79% (19/24)	yes[a]	1 year
Colombo et al, 2004 [40]	100% (27/27)	yes[a]	≤ 1 year
Muto et al, 2004 [41]	95% (58/61)	yes[a]	≤ 6 months
Terrone, Rosetti et al, 2004 [42]	93% (26/28)	yes[a]	≤ 2 months
Kessler, Studer et al, 2004 [2]	60% (38)[b]	bilateral	≤ 2 years[b]
	33% (218)[b]	unilateral	
	13% (75)[b]	no	
Zippe et al, 2004 [37]	50% (8/16)	yes	≥ 1 year
	3% (1/33)	no	

[a] Prostate sparing.
[b] Kaplan-Meier method.

sparing cystectomy technique and younger age were independently associated with more frequent recovery of erectile function (Table 1). Furthermore, bilateral preservation of the neurovascular bundles gave the best results (Fig. 7). However, data regarding preoperative erectile function were not available, and postoperative erectile function was assessed by questionnaire, but not by a validated sexual function questionnaire. Zippe et al [37] investigated sexual dysfunction in men after radical cystectomy using the validated abridged five-item International Index of Erectile function and found that only 9 (14%) of 49 sexually active men were potent after surgery. Fifty percent of the men with nerve-sparing surgery remained potent, whereas only 3% of the men without nerve sparing retained sexual function.

Several authors reported excellent results regarding sexual function with a seminal vesicle and prostate sparing cystectomy [5,38–42]. If prostate-sparing cystectomy with subsequent orthotopic bladder substitution is attempted, then preoperative TUR-P (to exclude transitional cell carcinoma) or adenoma enucleation during cystectomy is mandatory to avoid outlet obstruction by prostatic tissue and subsequent post void residuals.

Although the results of prostate-sparing cystectomy in carefully selected patients suggest no adverse effects on cancer management, further experience especially in the long term is required before recommending this type of procedure as a valid option in the management of muscle invasive or high grade, multifocal superficial bladder cancer.

In the female, data concerning the effect of radical cystectomy on sexual function is rare. Volkmer et al [43] reported that all aspects of female sexuality may remain unchanged following non–nerve-sparing cystectomy and ileal orthotopic bladder substitution as long as sexual activity is not impaired for other reasons. However, these results are hampered by the retrospective study design where preoperative sexual function was evaluated 1 to 17 years following cystectomy. In a recent prospective investigation [44] using the Index of Female Sexual Function questionnaire only about half of the 27 patients were able to have successful vaginal intercourse following non–nerve-sparing radical cystectomy. The most common symptoms reported by these patients included diminished sexual desire, decreased vaginal lubrication, dyspareunia, and

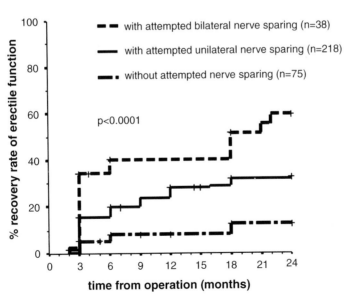

Fig. 7. After radical cystoprostatectomy and ileal orthotopic bladder substitution, patients with attempted bi- or unilateral nerve sparing had a significantly higher recovery rate of erectile function compared with those without attempted nerve sparing. However, it should be considered that when applying the Kaplan-Meier method patients reporting recovery of erectile function remain classified as potent even if they become impotent later on. (*From* Kessler TM, Burkhard FC, Perimenis P, et al. Attempted nerve sparing surgery and age have a significant effect on urinary continence and erectile function after radical cystoprostatectomy and ileal orthotopic bladder substitution. J Urol 2004;172:1323–7; with permission.)

diminished ability or inability to achieve orgasm. This could be due to a non–nerve-sparing technique because autonomic nerve damage may result in insufficient lubrication causing vaginal dryness and dyspareunia [45].

Summary

The autonomic sympathetic and parasympathetic nerve fibers from the pelvic plexus pass through the dorsomedial pedicle of the bladder ending as the paraprostatic neurovascular bundle or paravaginal plexus before supplying the urogenital diaphragm, sphincter, and erectile organs. Preservation of the autonomic innervation is important for sexual, lower urinary tract, and bowel function. Oncologic outcome is not compromised by a nerve-sparing cystectomy if adequate selection criteria are applied. During pelvic lymphadenectomy nerve sparing is not impaired as long as the dissection is performed on the lateral, not medial side of the ureters, where the nerves lie. Nerve-sparing radical cystectomy preserves sexual function and, in the case of orthotopic bladder substitution, better continence, and decreased catheterization rates (especially in women) are achieved. Therefore, under the proper circumstances, nerve-sparing radical cystectomy is to be strongly recommended.

References

[1] Turner WH, Danuser H, Moehrle K, et al. The effect of nerve sparing cystectomy technique on postoperative continence after orthotopic bladder substitution. J Urol 1997;158:2118–22.

[2] Kessler TM, Burkhard FC, Perimenis P, et al. Attempted nerve sparing surgery and age have a significant effect on urinary continence and erectile function after radical cystoprostatectomy and ileal orthotopic bladder substitution. J Urol 2004;172:1323–7.

[3] Brendler CB, Steinberg GD, Marshall FF, et al. Local recurrence and survival following nerve-sparing radical cystoprostatectomy. J Urol 1990; 144:1137–40 (discussion 1140–1).

[4] Schoenberg MP, Walsh PC, Breazeale DR, et al. Local recurrence and survival following nerve sparing radical cystoprostatectomy for bladder cancer: 10-year followup. J Urol 1996;155:490–4.

[5] Vallancien G, Abou El Fettouh H, Cathelineau X, et al. Cystectomy with prostate sparing for bladder cancer in 100 patients: 10-year experience. J Urol 2002;168:2413–7.

[6] Akita K, Sakamoto H, Sato T. Origins and courses of the nervous branches to the male urethral sphinc-

ter. Surg Radiol Anat 2003;25:387–92 (Epub 2003 Sep 6).

[7] Yucel S, De Souza A Jr, Baskin LS. Neuroanatomy of the human female lower urogenital tract. J Urol 2004;172:191–5.

[8] Zvara P, Carrier S, Kour NW, et al. The detailed neuroanatomy of the human striated urethral sphincter. Br J Urol 1994;74:182–7.

[9] Nelson CP, Montie JE, McGuire EJ, et al. Intraoperative nerve stimulation with measurement of urethral sphincter pressure changes during radical retropubic prostatectomy: a feasibility study. J Urol 2003;169:2225–8.

[10] Hugonnet CL, Danuser H, Springer JP, et al. Urethral sensitivity and the impact on urinary continence in patients with an ileal bladder substitute after cystectomy. J Urol 2001;165:1502–5.

[11] Gulati N, Kumar VJ, Barsaul M, et al. Urodynamic profile after Wertheim's hysterectomy. Indian J Cancer 2001;38:96–102.

[12] Hübner WA, Trigo-Rocha F, Plas EG, et al. Functional bladder replacement after radical cystectomy in the female: experimental investigation of a new concept. Eur Urol 1993;23:400–4.

[13] Strasser H, Ninkovic M, Hess M, et al. Anatomic and functional studies of the male and female urethral sphincter. World J Urol 2000;18:324–9.

[14] Doherty A, Burkhard F, Holliger S, et al. Bladder substitution in women. Curr Urol Rep 2001;2: 350–6.

[15] Ottesen B, Fahrenkrug J. Vasoactive intestinal polypeptide and other preprovasoactive intestinal polypeptide-derived peptides in the female and male genital tract: localization, biosynthesis, and functional and clinical significance. Am J Obstet Gynecol 1995;172:1615–31.

[16] Litwin MS, Sadetsky N, Pasta DJ, et al. Bowel function and bother after treatment for early stage prostate cancer: a longitudinal quality of life analysis from CaPSURE. J Urol 2004;172:515–9.

[17] Gralnek D, Wessells H, Cui H, et al. Differences in sexual function and quality of life after nerve sparing and nonnerve sparing radical retropubic prostatectomy. J Urol 2000;163:1166–9 (discussion 1169–70).

[18] Skinner DG. Management of invasive bladder cancer: a meticulous pelvic node dissection can make a difference. J Urol 1982;128:34–6.

[19] Thalmann GN, Fleischmann A, Mills RD, et al. Lymphadenectomy in bladder cancer. EAU Update Series 2003;1:100–7.

[20] Abol-Enein H, El-Baz M, Abd El-Hameed MA, et al. Lymph node involvement in patients with bladder cancer treated with radical cystectomy: a pathoanatomical study—a single center experience. J Urol 2004;172:1818–21.

[21] Burkhard FC, Studer UE. Orthotopic urinary diversion using an ileal low-pressure bladder substitute with an afferent tubular segment. Atlas Urol Clin North Am 2001;9:57–73.

[22] Madersbacher S, Hochreiter W, Burkhard F, et al. Radical cystectomy for bladder cancer today—a homogeneous series without neoadjuvant therapy. J Clin Oncol 2003;21:690–6.

[23] Stein JP, Lieskovsky G, Cote R, et al. Radical cystectomy in the treatment of invasive bladder cancer: long-term results in 1,054 patients. J Clin Oncol 2001;19:666–75.

[24] Hautmann RE, de Petriconi R, Gottfried HW, et al. The ileal neobladder: complications and functional results in 363 patients after 11 years of followup. J Urol 1999;161:422–7 (discussion 427–8).

[25] Abol-Enein H, Ghoneim MA. Functional results of orthotopic ileal neobladder with serous-lined extramural ureteral reimplantation: experience with 450 patients. J Urol 2001;165:1427–32.

[26] Stein JP, Dunn MD, Quek ML, et al. The orthotopic T pouch ileal neobladder: experience with 209 patients. J Urol 2004;172:584–7.

[27] Mills RD, Studer UE. Female orthotopic bladder substitution: a good operation in the right circumstances. J Urol 2000;163:1501–4.

[28] Ali-El-Dein B, Gomha M, Ghoneim MA. Critical evaluation of the problem of chronic urinary retention after orthotopic bladder substitution in women. J Urol 2002;168:587–92.

[29] Lee CT, Hafez KS, Sheffield JH, et al. Orthotopic bladder substitution in women: nontraditional applications. J Urol 2004;171:1585–8.

[30] Stenzl A, Jarolim L, Coloby P, et al. Urethra-sparing cystectomy and orthotopic urinary diversion in women with malignant pelvic tumors. Cancer 2001; 92:1864–71.

[31] Oelrich TM. The striated urogenital sphincter muscle in the female. Anat Rec 1983;205:223–32.

[32] Hammerer P, Michl U, Meyer-Moldenhauer WH, et al. Urethral closure pressure changes with age in men. J Urol 1996;156:1741–3.

[33] Gilpin SA, Gilpin CJ, Dixon JS, et al. The effect of age on the autonomic innervation of the urinary bladder. Br J Urol 1986;58:378–81.

[34] Hautmann RE. Urinary diversion: ileal conduit to neobladder. J Urol 2003;169:834–42.

[35] Studer UE, Turner WH. The ileal orthotopic bladder. Urology 1995;45:185–9.

[36] Studer UE, Zingg EJ. Ileal orthotopic bladder substitutes. What we have learned from 12 years' experience with 200 patients. Urol Clin North Am 1997; 24:781–93.

[37] Zippe CD, Raina R, Massanyi EZ, et al. Sexual function after male radical cystectomy in a sexually active population. Urology 2004;64:682–5 (discussion 685–6).

[38] Spitz A, Stein JP, Lieskovsky G, et al. Orthotopic urinary diversion with preservation of erectile and ejaculatory function in men requiring radical cystectomy for nonurothelial malignancy: a new technique. J Urol 1999;161:1761–4.

[39] Meinhardt W, Horenblas S. Sexuality preserving cystectomy and neobladder (SPCN): functional results of a neobladder anastomosed to the prostate. Eur Urol 2003;43:646–50.

[40] Colombo R, Bertini R, Salonia A, et al. Overall clinical outcomes after nerve and seminal sparing radical cystectomy for the treatment of organ confined bladder cancer. J Urol 2004;171:1819–22 (discussion 1822).

[41] Muto G, Bardari F, D'Urso L, et al. Seminal sparing cystectomy and ileocapsuloplasty: long-term followup results. J Urol 2004;172:76–80.

[42] Terrone C, Cracco C, Scarpa RM, et al. Supra-ampullar cystectomy with preservation of sexual function and ileal orthotopic reservoir for bladder tumor: twenty years of experience. Eur Urol 2004; 46:264–9 (discussion 269–70).

[43] Volkmer BG, Gschwend JE, Herkommer K, et al. Cystectomy and orthotopic ileal neobladder: the impact on female sexuality. J Urol 2004;172:2353–7.

[44] Zippe CD, Raina R, Shah AD, et al. Female sexual dysfunction after radical cystectomy: a new outcome measure. Urology 2004;63:1153–7.

[45] Keating JP. Sexual function after rectal excision. ANZ J Surg 2004;74:248–59.

ELSEVIER
SAUNDERS

Urol Clin N Am 32 (2005) 177–185

**UROLOGIC
CLINICS
of North America**

Neobladder with Prostatic Capsule and Seminal-sparing Cystectomy for Bladder Cancer: A Step in the Wrong Direction

Richard E. Hautmann, MD[a],*, John P. Stein, MD, FACS[b]

[a]*Department of Urology, University of Ulm, Prittwitzstrasse 43, Ulm D-89075, Germany*
[b]*Department of Urology, USC/Norris Cancer Center, 1441 Eastlake Avenue,
Suite 7416, Los Angeles, CA 90089-9178, USA*

The initial intent of bladder replacement procedures was not to improve survival or prognosis, or to decrease renal and metabolic complications, but rather to improve the quality of life. The success of total bladder substitution largely depends on the degree of continence that the patient is able to achieve. Although good daytime continence was reported with most techniques, some patients had a high voiding frequency and occasionally were wet at night, unless they voided more frequently or used a collection device.

Preservation of apical prostatic tissue or the prostatic capsule for anastomosis with a reservoir has been suggested by several authors to improve urinary continence at a time when orthotopic reconstruction was experimental surgery and the currently used technical principles of neobladders were unknown [1–5]. It was assumed that preservation of the prostatic apex would improve urinary continence in orthotopic reservoirs based on the following rationale: this part of a prostate contains the inner smooth muscle component of a distal urethral sphincteric mechanism [6], which presumably augments the external striated muscle component in maintaining continence. Theoretically, continence in these patients would be better than in those with complete resection of the prostate.

Complete removal of the prostate versus partial preservation can be considered from three aspects: (1) the possibility of violating the principles of oncologic surgery, (2) the effects on continence, and (3) the effect on sexuality. This article analyzes recent results in sexual function preserving cystectomy, including indications, risks, and outcome.

Patient selection

The literature does not specify criteria for sexuality-preserving cystectomy. Several studies report patient characteristics and outcome (Table 1). The indication for surgery used by Spitz et al [7] was bladder signet ring carcinoma, bladder leiomyosarcoma, and extensive polypoid cystitis glandularis refractory to conservative and transurethral management. These authors excluded urothelial carcinoma because they strongly believed this was contraindicated in the sexuality-preserving procedure, and that is why their data are not included in this article. Colombo et al [8] initially reserved seminal-sparing surgery for patients with aggressive superficial disease (Ta, T1, or carcinoma in situ). All patients in this series had multifocal disease, multiple recurrences, short disease-free intervals, and grade progression despite intravesical therapy. A later study by the same group subsequently extended the indication to patients with muscle-invasive, but organ-confined disease (T2 a-b) [9]. Muto et al [10] performed seminal vesical-sparing cystectomy in patients with superficial disease (Ta-T1, G2-G3) in 55 and invasive bladder cancer (T2 a-b, G3) in 5 of 61 patients, respectively. They excluded

---

* Corresponding author.
E-mail address: richard.hautmann@medizin.
uni-ulm.de (R.E. Hautmann).

Table 1
Sexual-function–preserving cystectomy: patient characteristics and follow-up

Author	Publ./Year	Patients		Follow-up (mo)	Tumor stage		Failure		Prostate cancer
		N	Mean age (y)		≤pT1 G3 pN0	pT2a-b pN0 M0	Local	Distant	
Botto et al [13]	BJU Int 2004	34	61	26	6/34	16/34	1/22	4/22	1/22
Muto et al [10]	J Urol 2004	61	49	68	55/61	5/61	0/60	6/60	1/61, 3 PIN 3/61
Colombo et al [9]	J Urol 2004	27	52	32	21/27	5/27	0/26	0/26	0/27
Vallancien et al [12]	J Urol 2002	100	64	38	22/62	40/62	3/62	14/62	3/100
Abuzeid [15]	J Urol 2005 [A]	45	30–48	NA	0/45	45/45	3/45	4/45	NA
Min et al [16]	J Urol 2005 [A]	12	19–56	34	12/12	0/12	0/12	2/12	NA
Terrone et al [14]	Eur Urol 2004	27	51	90	23/25	2/25	0/25	4/25	0/25
Total		306			139/266	113/266	7/252	34/252	5/235

Abbreviation: NA, not available.

patients with invasive tumors close to the bladder neck or with multifocal invasive disease. Horenblas et al [11] were the only group to include a patient with T3 G3 N1 M0 bladder cancer, along with female patients. Their data have not been included in this article. Patients with involvement of bladder neck, prostatic urethra, or prostatic stroma are absolutely considered inappropriate for this type of operation [11,12].

Although coexisting prostate cancer is unanimously considered a contraindication for sexuality-preserving cystectomy, screening procedures vary. Spitz et al [7] excluded patients at moderate or high risk of prostate cancer, but they did not screen their sample because their oldest patient was just 49 years old and the median age of the cohort was 26. Colombo et al [8] in their first series (age 36–48 years) determined prostate-specific antigen (PSA) preoperatively followed by pathologic examination of the transurethral resection (TUR) chips obtained at the TUR of the prostate before cystectomy. In a second study, this group included patients up to 61 years. Only patients with normal findings on digital rectal examination (DRE), total serum PSA less than 4 ng/mL, and a free-to-total PSA ratio greater than 25% were included. In 2001, they added transrectal ultrasound (TRUS)-guided prostate biopsy in all patients, regardless of DRE or PSA results [9]. They identified one patient with prostate cancer by transurethral resection of the prostate (TURP) pathology. Muto et al [10] using PSA, DRE, and TRUS of the prostate without biopsy reported a 4.9% incidence (three cases) of high-grade prostate intraepithelial neoplasia and a 1.9% incidence (one case) of prostate cancer. Vallancien et al [12] excluded prostate cancer preoperatively by normal DRE, PSA of less than 4 ng/mL, and a normal TRUS. Later, they added a PSA ratio of greater than 15% with normal prostate biopsy findings in cases of suspected prostate cancer. As many as 57 (39%) of their 165 cystectomy patients were excluded preoperatively using this algorithm. This group performed frozen sections of the TURP material on their 100 patients; three cases of prostate cancer were diagnosed postoperatively (two pathologic errors and one de novo within 5 years follow-up).

Botto et al [13] in their 34 patients used a TURP to exclude involvement of TCC of the prostate in all clinical less than T2 N0 M0 patients. The studies from Terrone et al [14], Abuzeid et al [15], and Min et al [16] are also included in this article (see Table 1).

Oncologic factors

Local recurrence and distant failure

In 139 (52%) of 266 patients with sexuality-preserving cystectomy reported in the literature a bladder cancer less than or equal to pT1 G3 N0 M0 was the indication for cystectomy. In another 113 (42%) of 266 patients a pT2 a-b N0 M0 tumor was the indication for cystectomy (see Table 1). The remaining 14 patients are not specified in the reports. The mean follow-up is approximately 40 months. In the authors' large radical cystoprostatectomy-only series at Ulm (N = 646), at a median follow-up of 36 months (range 0–218 months) was observed a 1.5% and 5.8% local recurrence rate for pTa/pTis/pT1, N0 M0 tumors, and pT2 a-b, N0 M0 tumors, respectively (Table 2). The distant failure rate at 36 months was 4.9% and 12.7% for pTa/pTis/pT1 and pT2 a-b, N0 M0, respectively. Based on the failure rates given stage by stage in Table 2 and the stage distribution of pTa/pTis/pT1 and pT2 a-b, N0 M0 in the combined sexuality-preserving cystectomy series (see Table 1), a maximum of 10 of 252 patients should have developed a local recurrence. A maximum of 21 of 252 patients in the sexuality-preserving should have had distant (metastatic) failure. The observed distant failure rate following sexuality-sparing cystectomy, after an average follow up of 40 months, however, is almost twice as high (34 of 252). This 14% distant failure rate is comparable with the distant failure rate for locally advanced, extravesical pT3 a-b, N0 M0 (18%) tumors (see Table 2).

Despite careful patient selection and exclusion of approximately 40% of patients because of oncologic reasons [12,13], the cancer outcome

Table 2
Pattern of recurrence in 646 patients with lymph node–negative TCC treated by radical cystoprostatectomy only at the Department of Urology, University of Ulm, from 1986 to 2003[a]

	N	Local failure N	Local failure %	Distant failure N	Distant failure %	Urinary tract recurrence N	Urinary tract recurrence %
pTa/is/1	203	3	1.5	10	4.9	12	5.9
pT2a-b	292	17	5.8	37	12.7	8	2.7
pT3a-b	105	13	12.4	19	18.1	3	2.9
pT4a-b	46	11	23.9	10	21.7	2	4.3
Total	646	44	6.8	76	11.8	25	3.9

Abbreviation: TCC, transitional-cell carcinoma.
[a] Surgery-only series.

following sexuality-preserving cystectomy is significantly worse than results obtained with standard radical cystoprostatectomy. Furthermore, the pattern of failure (local versus distant) is different from standard radical cystectomy series. With only seven observed local failures following sexuality-preserving cystectomy almost all of the 34 distant failures developed without local recurrence. This probably reflects the result of direct tumor spill to liver and lungs without passing the regional lymph nodes. The authors agree with the hypotheses forwarded by Botto et al [13]: metastatic diffusion could have started or occurred during the prostate resection 2 weeks before cystectomy. The prostate was resected in patients whose urine contained urothelial bladder cells, and prostate vessels opened during resection could have been a route for tumor-cell dissemination and a starting point for hematogenous metastasis. Furthermore, during sexuality-preserving cystectomy, when the posterior plane is dissected, sparing the prostatic capsule and seminal vesicles, cancer cells could have subsequently escaped.

Prostate cancer

Most prostate cancers detected incidentally in the prostates of cystoprostatectomies performed for bladder carcinoma have been regarded as clinically insignificant. The reported incidence of prostate carcinoma in cystoprostatectomy specimens is approximately 40%, with approximately 20% of these tumors considered potentially clinically significant (Table 3) [17–21]. This relatively common involvement by prostate carcinoma (including clinically insignificant prostate carcinomas) has been argued to support removing all prostate tissue as part of standard cystoprostatectomy. Anatomic location of such prostate carcinoma, however, specifically apical involvement, has only rarely been described [18].

In a recent study, Revelo et al [17] addressed the incidence and location of prostate carcinoma in prostates from cystoprostatectomy specimens removed for transitional-cell carcinoma (TCC) in regard for possible apical-sparing surgery. In this study [17] of 121 prostates, 50 (41%) had unsuspected prostate carcinoma, of which 24 (48%) were clinically significant. Importantly, of prostatic carcinomas, 30 (60%) of 50 involved the apex, including 19 (79%) of 24 that were significant. Their frequency of extracapsular extension

Table 3

Incidence of prostate carcinoma in cystoprostatectomy specimens

Reference	Total no.	Median age (y)	% PCA	Step-section
Kabalin et al [18]	66	64	38	Yes (3 mm)
Montie et al [19]	84	64	46	Yes (4–5 mm)
Revelo et al [17]	121	67	41	Yes (2–3 mm)
Stein et al [20]	843	67	29	No
Hautmann et al [21]	133	60	44	Yes (3 mm)

Abbreviation: PCA, prostate cancer.

(16%) and Gleason patterns 4 and 5 (score 7 or greater, 20%) were also higher than noted previously (eg, 3%–10% and 11%, respectively) [18,19,22,23], further supporting the validity of this result.

In the cystoprostatectomy series of Moutzouris et al [24], 16 cases with prostatic carcinoma had apical involvement by prostate carcinoma, of which all had pathology parameters suggesting that they were clinically insignificant [24]. This group concluded that apical involvement by prostate carcinoma should warrant complete prostate resection [25]. In the study by Revelo et al [17], clinically insignificant or clinically significant prostate carcinoma involved the prostatic apex in approximately 25% of cases overall, with approximately two thirds being so-called "clinically significant."

In a recent study Hautmann et al [21] addressed the probability of overlooking clinically significant prostate cancer using sextant biopsy. They analyzed specimens from 133 consecutive patients (mean age of 60 years) undergoing cystoprostatectomy for bladder cancer. Patients were included in the study if they had a serum PSA less than 4 ng/mL, a normal DRE before surgery, and a free PSA of greater than 25%. A total of 151 consecutive men with prostate carcinoma served as a control. Systematic sextant biopsy or rebiopsy was done in the operating room immediately following cystoprostatectomy or radical prostatectomy, respectively. All prostate specimens were step sectioned (3 mm). The threshold defined to distinguish between significant and insignificant cancer was 0.5 cm^3. The authors found that specimen biopsy can well

simulate transrectal prostate biopsy. Incidental prostate cancer was found in 58 (44%) of the 133 bladder cancer patients. Tumor volume was 0.5 cm^3 or less in 47 cases. Sextant biopsy detected seven cancers, including 4 (9%) of 47 that were insignificant and 3 (27%) of 11 that were clinically significant. Fine-needle aspiration cytology also detected seven cancers, including three (6%) and four (36%) that were insignificant and significant, respectively. Sextant biopsy missed 8 (73%) of 11 of significant prostate cancer. Three quarters of all tumors were Gleason $3 + 3 = 6$. Four of the significant cancers had Gleason patterns 4 and 5. The data suggest that despite careful screening for sexuality-preserving cystectomy, it is likely to miss a significant prostate cancer in 6% of patients. In the 235 cases with sexuality-sparing cystectomy reported in the literature (see Table 1), five cases with prostatic carcinoma and three with high-grade prostate intraepithelial neoplasia have been reported. The follow-up of all the reported series, however, is still too limited to asses the true clinical impact regarding prostate cancer after different types of surgical procedures of the prostate.

TCC in prostate

An important consideration for prostatic apical sparing during cystoprostatectomy is the extent or location of TCC in the prostate. The reported incidence of TCC involving the prostate in association with bladder TCC is 17% to 48% (Table 4) [26]. Revelo et al [17] in a series using totally submitted prostates and including careful evaluation of the prostatic urethra and periurethral ducts for urothelial carcinoma in situ or severe dysplasia found that 48% of the prostates from cystoprostatectomy specimens were involved by TCC. Most of these cases were those with urothelial carcinoma in situ or severe dysplasia of the prostatic urethra. In contrast to prostate cancer, however, apical involvement by TCC was less common, being present in only 19 (16%) of the 121 patients. Importantly, when apical involvement was present (either by invasive TCC or urethral-periurethral duct urothelial carcinoma in situ, neither of which is appropriate to "leave-in"), it was universally associated with disease located in the more proximal prostate. This raises serious oncologic concerns regarding preservation of the prostate in patients with TCC. Vallancien et al [12] reported a rate of only 2% for

Table 4
TCC in prostates from cystoprostatectomies for bladder cancer

Reference	Total no.	Prostate TCC (%)	Ducts or urethra (%)	Invasive (stroma) (%)	Step-section
Reese et al [26]	115	33 (29)	17 (15)	16 (14)	Yes
Wood et al [25]	84	36 (43)	22 (26)	14 (17)	Yes
Revelo et al [17]	121	58 (48)	45 (37)	13 (10)	Yes

Abbreviation: TCC, transitional-cell carcinoma.

recurrent urothelial cancer in the prostatic fossa after a mean follow-up of 38 months.

Functional outcomes

Daytime-nighttime continence

The improvement in quality of life after orthotopic bladder substitution compared with alternative forms of diversion fails to be achieved when voiding dysfunction arises. Some degree of nocturnal leakage is a constant finding in most reports despite a technically sound operation. Nocturnal incontinence after orthotopic reconstruction is more common, lasts longer than daytime incontinence, and is a feature shared by all forms of neobladder. Nocturnal enuresis may develop in almost 28% of patients (range 0%–67%) [27]. Table 5 presents the daytime and nighttime continence data of several large radical cystectomy series from centers of excellence [28–32]. In a review of 2238 patients Steers [27] found a daytime continence rate of 87% and a nighttime continence rate of 72%.

The primary goal of prostate-sparing cystectomy for bladder cancer is to minimize the risk of incontinence and impotence. Table 6 presents data that are frequently used to support this concept [7–12,33].

Colombo et al [9] reported immediate continence after catheter removal in 67% of patients and in 100% after 15 days. The mean interval between voids was 2.4 hours at 3 months and 3.5 hours at 12 months. Urodynamic evaluation revealed adequate neobladder volume (mean 430 mL); low filling pressure; and high urethral pressure. Fifteen percent of patients had bladder outlet obstruction requiring endoscopic treatment, mainly caused by folds of ileal mucosa obstructing the bladder outlet. Muto et al [10] reported daytime continence in 95% of patients but nighttime continence in just 31%. One of their patients required continuous intermittent catheterization for large residuals. Vallancien et al [12] reported 97% daytime and 95% nighttime continence with nocturia frequency of one to three times. None of the patients required continuous intermittent catheterization. In a urodynamic study of voiding patterns after prostate-sparing surgery, Meinhardt and Horenblas [33] noted that only a minority of patients start voiding by pelvic floor relaxation followed by a pressure rise in the neobladder. Most patients start with a Valsalva's maneuver and strain to complete micturition. International Prostate Symptom Score (IPSS) scores were higher postoperatively, mainly because of loss of the detrusor contractile effect and a need to strain to empty.

Table 7 presents another seven series of sexual function–preserving cystectomy that have been either overlooked (eg, Koraitim et al [34]) or are brand new [13–16,35,36]. These studies present inconsistent and contradictory clinical outcomes, the functional results of which are equal to or even worse than following standard cystectomy.

Table 5
Continence rates following radical cystoprostatectomy and neobladder formation

Group	No. of patients	Age (y)	Diversion	% Continence Day	Night
Shaaban et al [28]	205	49	W-pouch	94	68
Steven and Poulsen [29]	166	62	Kock	97	94
Madersbacher et al [30]	176	63	Studer	92	82
Hautmann et al [31]	290	63	W-pouch	84	83
Stein et al [32]	209	69	T-pouch	87	72

Table 6
Sexual function–preserving cystectomy: functional results

| Author | No. | Continence (%) | | Sexual function (%) | | | |
		Day	Night	Potency	Antegrade	Retrograde	Mixed
Spitz et al [7]	4	100	100	100	75	25	0
Muto et al [10]	61	95	31	95	0	100	0
Vallancien et al [12]	100	97	95	82	0	100	0
Horenblas et al [11,33]	24	96	87.5	85[a]	50[a]	40[a]	10[a]
Colombo et al [8,9]	27	100	100	100	11.1	81.5	7.4

[a] In 20 out of 24 sexually active men.

Functional outcomes

Sexual function

The greatest potential advantage of prostatic capsule and seminal-sparing cystectomy, is preservation of sexual function. Table 6 presents the data of the frequently discussed series.

An age limit for sexuality-preserving cystectomy has never been proposed. Initially some authors included only patients under age 50. Encouraging results prompted them to include sexually active patients of all ages who were interested in postoperative sexual function [12]. To date the oldest reported patient was 82 years at the time of surgery. An optimal preoperative evaluation of sexual function has not been established [8,11]. Horenblas et al [11] used a structured interview on erection and ejaculation and nightly

RigiScan, whereas Colombo et al [9] used the International Index of Erectile Function (IIEF) questionnaire with the addition of several global assessment questions, combined with RigiScan and dynamic penile power ultrasound.

Sexual function includes several domains (sexual satisfaction, erection, ejaculation, and fertility), and its preservation is of major concern to sexual active men regardless of age. The published results of erectile function preservation following modified cystectomy are indeed encouraging (see Tables 6 and 7). All patients studied by Colombo et al [8,9] reported rapid return of erections and satisfactory sexual performance postoperatively. In all cases, IIEF scores, RigiScan test, and sonographic penile hemodynamics were normal. Spitz et al [7] reported immediate return of erections in their young patients. Muto et al [10]

Table 7
Sexual function–preserving cystectomy: functional results

| Author | No. | Continence (%) | | Sexual function (%) | | | |
		Day	Night	Potency	Antegrade	Retrograde	Mixed
Min et al [16]	32	97	88	91			
Dall'Oglio et al [36]	22	85	38	36			
Burday et al [35]							
Apex	17	65	30	58.8			
Prostate	6			100			
NV bundle	12	58	42	20			
Botto et al [13]	27	80	80	90	100		
Koraitim et al [34]							
Apex	13	100	70	NA			
Urethra	25	88	40	NA			
Abuzeid [15]							
Prostate	20	100 CIC	100 CIC	95			
Genital		100	100	88	72		
Terrone et al [14]	27	60; 20 CIC		93	54		

Abbreviations: CIC, continuous intermittent catheterization; NA, not applicable; NV, neurovascular.

reported nighttime erections 8 to 10 days post-operatively in 80% of patients and normal sexual function 1 to 2 months postoperatively in 90% of patients. In 5% of patients, erection recovered after 6 months and in another 5% there were no spontaneous erections and intracavernous injection of alprostadil was required. Horenblas et al [11] reported spontaneous erections in 7 out of 10 patients and erections with the use of sildenafil in two. Vallancien et al [12] reported intact potency in 82% of patients.

The ejaculation data are presented in Tables 6 and 7. All eight patients studied by Colombo et al [8,9] had retrograde ejaculation, and four had partial antegrade ejaculation. Sperm retrieval from the antegrade ejaculate showed low volume and count, and sperm retrieved from urine by catheterization following masturbation showed an average count of 8×10^6 sperms/mL and a motility of 20% to 50%. None of their patients, however, attempted to achieve pregnancy. Three of the patients described by Spitz et al [7] maintained antegrade ejaculation; one had a retrograde ejaculation. There was a steady improvement in postoperative ejaculate volume and sperm count, and one patient fathered a child 1 year later. This is the only documented case of fertility and spontaneous conception following sexuality-sparing cystectomy. Horenblas et al [11] reported antegrade ejaculation in five patients, retrograde in four, and intermittent antegrade-retrograde in one. In the series of Muto et al. [10] and Vallancien et al [12], postoperative retrograde ejaculation was the rule. Antegrade ejaculation seems to be more common in patients who do not have TURP or adenoma enucleation.

The newer and not widely acknowledged articles from Table 7 present data on sexual function that are clearly inferior to those of Table 6, but still better than after standard cystectomy and only slightly better than after nerve-sparing cystectomy [37,38].

Recently, van Cangh et al [39] reported their functional results and quality of life 10 years following radical prostatectomy. Interestingly, 87% of patients have no or little sexual activity, which is not statistically different from controls (86%). In this cohort of patients, who underwent radical prostatectomy 10 years prior (mean present age 75), erectile dysfunction, strongly contrasting with incontinence, does not impact overall quality of life. They conclude that quality of life is preserved 10 years after surgery, except in a small portion of patients with persisting severe

incontinence. Erectile dysfunction, however, seems to be of less concern over time.

Summary

A laudable trend in urologic surgical oncology is to minimize operative morbidity by anatomic and functional organ preservation without compromising radicality. An increasing number of authors have taken advantage of the sexual-function–preserving cystectomy for bladder cancer. The modified procedure includes cystectomy with sparing of prostate, vasa deferens, seminal vesicles, and resection of a prostatic adenoma to avoid bladder outlet obstruction and bladder reconstruction with an orthotopic reservoir. This article focuses on studies from the last 15 years and includes the results from 13 centers worldwide. Many of them report a pattern of failure (local versus distant) that is highly unusual. Although a local recurrence rate of 7 of 252 patients is to be expected in this combined series the distant failure rate of 34 of 252 patients is at least twice as high as expected for the given series of superficial or organ-confined TCC. The observed distant failure rate of sexuality-preserving cystectomy in this potentially lethal disease is more than 5% higher as compared with standard radical cystectomy. The precise underlying mechanism of this unexpected pattern of failure following sexuality-sparing cystectomy is not fully understood. Furthermore, surgeons considering procedures that preserve a portion of the prostatic urethra, the prostatic capsule, or the entire prostate should recognize a 6% risk of significant prostatic cancer in any residual tissue, and the potential risk of urethral tumor involvement with TCC.

Daytime continence following radical versus sexuality-sparing cystectomy is identical. Data on nighttime continence of sexuality-sparing cystectomy are inconclusive. The continuous intermittent catheterization rate following sexuality-sparing cystectomy, however, seems to be higher than after standard cystectomy.

The only advantage sexuality-preserving cystectomy has is indeed preservation of these functions in a much higher percentage than following standard or nerve-sparing cystectomy. This is at the cost of radicality, however, and results in a 10% to 15% higher oncologic failure rate. Consequently, sexuality-sparing cystectomy for bladder cancer is a step in the wrong direction and should be abandoned.

References

[1] McDougal WS. Bladder reconstruction following cystectomy by uretero-ileocolourethrostomy. J Urol 1986;135:698–701.

[2] Steven K, Klarskov P, Jakobsen H, et al. Transpubic cystectomy and ileocecal replacement after preoperative radiotherapy for bladder cancer. J Urol 1986; 135:470–5.

[3] Zinman L, Libertino JA. Right colocystoplasty for bladder replacement. Urol Clin North Am 1986;13: 321–31.

[4] Lilien OM, Camey M. 25-year experience with replacement of the human bladder (Camey procedure). J Urol 1984;132:886–91.

[5] Schilling A, Friesen A. Transprostatic selective cystectomy with an ileal bladder. Eur Urol 1990;18: 253–7.

[6] Koraitim MM, Atta MA, Foda MK. Early and late cystometry of detubularized and non-detubularized intestinal neobladders: new observations and physiological correlates. J Urol 1995;154:1700–3.

[7] Spitz A, Stein JP, Lieskovsky G, et al. Orthotopic urinary diversion with preservation of erectile and ejaculatory function in men requiring radical cystectomy for nonurethelial malignancy: an new technique. J Urol 1999;161:1761–4.

[8] Colombo R, Bertini R, Salonia A, et al. Nerve and seminal sparing radical cystectomy with orthotopic urinary diversion for select patients with superficial bladder cancer: an innovative surgical approach. J Urol 2001;165:51–5.

[9] Colombo R, Bertini R, Salonia A, et al. Overall clinical outcomes after nerve and seminal sparing radical cystectomy for the treatment of organ confined bladder cancer. J Urol 2004;171:1819–22.

[10] Muto G, Bardari F, D'Urso L, et al. Seminal sparing cystectomy and ileocapsuloplasty: long-term follow-up results. J Urol 2004;172:76–80.

[11] Horenblas S, Meinhardt W, Ijzerman W, et al. Sexuality preserving cystectomy and neobladder: initial results. J Urol 2001;166:837–40.

[12] Vallancien G, Abou EF, Cathelineau X, et al. Cystectomy with prostate sparing for bladder cancer in 100 patients: 10-year experience. J Urol 2002;168: 2413–7.

[13] Botto H, Sebe P, Molinie V, et al. Prostatic capsule- and seminal-sparing cystectomy for bladder carcinoma: initial results for selected patients. BJU Int 2004;94:1021–5.

[14] Terrone C, Cracco C, Scarpa RM, et al. Supra-ampullar cystectomy with preservation of sexual function and ileal orthotopic reservoir for bladder tumor: twenty years of experience. Eur Urol 2004; 46:264–70.

[15] Abuzeid AM Jr, Saleem MDS, Badawy AA Jr, et al. Genital sparing radical cystectomy for organ confined bladder carcinoma: impact on tumor control

and quality of life. J Urol 2005;173A:05-AB-4215-AUA.

[16] Min Y, Wei-ming W, Ying-jian Z. Clinical outcomes of nerve and seminal sparing cystectomy for the treatment of malignant and nonmalignant bladder disease. J Urol 2005;173A:05-AB-4392-AUA.

[17] Revelo MP, Cookson MS, Chang SS, et al. Incidence and location of prostate and urothelial carcinoma in prostates from cystoprostatectomies: implications for possible apical sparing surgery. J Urol 2004;171:646–51.

[18] Kabalin JN, McNeal JE, Price HM, et al. Unsuspected adenocarcinoma of the prostate in patients undergoing cystoprostatectomy for other causes: incidence, histology and morphometric observations. J Urol 1989;141:1091.

[19] Montie JE, Wood DP Jr, Pontes JE, et al. Adenocarcinoma of the prostate in cystoprostatectomy specimens removed for bladder cancer. Cancer 1989;63: 381.

[20] Stein JP, et al. Incidence of PCA in radical cystectomy specimens for bladder cancer. J Clin Oncol 2001;19:666.

[21] Hautmann S, et al. Incidence of PCA in radical cystectomy specimens for bladder cancer. J Urol 2000; 163:1734–8.

[22] Stamey TA, Freiha FS, McNeal JE, et al. Localized prostate cancer. Relationship of tumor volume to clinical significance for treatment of prostate cancer. Cancer 1993;71:933.

[23] Ohori M, Wheeler TM, Dunn JK, et al. The pathological features und prognosis of prostate cancer detectable with current diagnostic tests. J Urol 1994; 152:1714.

[24] Moutzouris G, Barbatis C, Plastiras D, et al. Incidence and histological findings of unsuspected prostatic adenocarcinoma in radical cystoprostatectomy for transitional cell carcinoma of the bladder. Scand J Urol Nephrol 1999;33:27.

[25] Wood DP Jr, Moutie JE, Poules JE, et al. Incidence of TCC in the prostate of radical cystectomy specimens. J Urol 1989;141:346.

[26] Reese JH, Freiha FS, Gelb AB, et al. Transitional cell carcinoma of the prostate in patients undergoing radical cystoprostatectomy. J Urol 1992;147:92.

[27] Steers WD. Orthotopic neobladder: functional outcomes. World J Urol 2000;18:330.

[28] Shaaban AA, Mosbah A, El-Bahnasawy MS, et al. The urethral Kock pouch: long-term functional and oncological results in men. BJU Int 2003;92:429–35.

[29] Steven K, Poulsen AL. The orthotopic Kock ileal neobladder: functional results, urodynamic features, complications and survival in 166 men. J Urol 2000; 164:288–95.

[30] Madersbacher S, Möhrle K, Burkhard F, et al. Long-term voiding pattern of patients with ileal orthotopic bladder substitutes. J Urol 2002;167: 2052–7.

[31] Hautmann RE, de Petriconi R, Gottfried HW, et al. The ileal neobladder: complications and functional results in 363 patients after 11 years of follow-up. U Urol 1999;161:422–7.

[32] Stein JP, Dunn MD, Queck ML, et al. The orthotopic T pouch ileal neobladder: experience with 209 patients. J Urol 2004;172:584–7.

[33] Meinhardt W, Horenblas S. Sexuality preserving cystectomy and neobladder (SPCN): functional results of a neobladder anastomosed to the prostate. Eur Urol 2003;43:646–50.

[34] Koraitim MM, Atta MA, Foda MK. Impact of the prostatic apex on continence and urinary flow in patients with intestinal neobladders. Brit J Urol 1996;78:534–6.

[35] Burday D, Weber T, Thurman S, et al. Prostate-sparing radical cystectomy: erectile function and continence. J Urol 2005;173A:05-AB-6128-AUA.

[36] Dall'Oglio MF, Crippa A, Antunes AA, et al. Can the radical cysto-adenomectomy preserve the post-operative sexual function and urinary continence rates after surgery? J Urol 2005;173A:05-AB-4875-AUA.

[37] Schoenberg MP, Walsh PC, Breazeale DR, et al. Local recurrence and survival following nerve sparing radical cystoprostatectomy for bladder cancer: 10-year follow-up. J Urol 1996;155:490–4.

[38] Brendler CB, Steinberg GD, Marshall FF, et al. Local recurrence and survival following nerve-sparing radical cystoprostatectomy. J Urol 1990;144:1131–41.

[39] Van Cangh PJ, Lion B, Tombal B. Functional results and quality of life 10 years after radical prostatectomy. Presented at the 3rd meeting of the AAEU. Milan, Italy, December 9–11, 2004.

ELSEVIER
SAUNDERS

Urol Clin N Am 32 (2005) 187–197

UROLOGIC
CLINICS
of North America

The Role of Lymphadenectomy in High-grade Invasive Bladder Cancer

John P. Stein, MD, FACS*, Donald G. Skinner, MD

Department of Urology, Norris Comprehensive Cancer Center, University of Southern California Keck School of Medicine, MS #74, 1441 Eastlake Avenue, Suite 7416, Los Angeles, CA 90089, USA

In the United States, bladder cancer is the fourth most common cancer in men and the eighth most common cancer in women, with transitional cell carcinoma (TCC) comprising nearly 90% of all primary bladder tumors. In 2004, it was estimated that 60,250 new patients would be diagnosed with bladder cancer, with 12,710 deaths from this disease [1]. Although most patients with bladder cancer present with superficial bladder tumors, 20% to 40% of patients present with or subsequently develop muscle invasive disease. Despite an early and aggressive approach toward high-grade invasive bladder cancer [2], nearly 25% of patients demonstrate pathologic evidence of lymph node metastases at the time of cystectomy [3–9]. These data suggest that a significant number of patients at the time of definitive therapy have locally advanced metastases to the regional lymph nodes.

The role of lymphadenectomy in genitourinary tumors has gained recent attention. There is little debate regarding the benefits of a lymph node dissection in testis tumors and penile cancer. Evidence also supports the concept of lymph node dissection in patients undergoing radical prostatectomy for prostate cancer [10] and radical nephrectomy for renal cell carcinoma [11]. Lymph node dissection also seems to be an important component in patients with high-grade invasive bladder cancer undergoing cystectomy. The rationale is a result of the natural history of the disease. Invasive bladder tumors tend to invade progressively from their superficial origin in the

mucosa to the lamina propria and sequentially into the muscularis propria, perivesical fat, and contiguous pelvic organs, with an increasing incidence of lymph node involvement at each site. This review evaluates historical and contemporary aspects of the role of lymphadenectomy in patients undergoing radical cystectomy for high-grade invasive TCC of the bladder.

A historical perspective

The role of lymphadenectomy in the treatment of bladder cancer has evolved over the past several decades. The initial belief regarding advanced bladder cancer with gross lymphadenopathy was that it was a uniformly fatal disease beyond the limits of surgical intervention. This notion was first challenged by Colston and Leadbetter in 1936 following the completion of an autopsy study of 98 patients with bladder cancer [12]. In that series, a significant number of bladder cancer cadavers were identified with limited metastatic disease restricted to the pelvic lymph nodes that was thought to be potentially amenable to surgical resection. A decade later, Jewett and Strong published similar findings in another autopsy series of 107 cases in which a percentage of cadavers with extravesical bladder tumors demonstrated metastatic involvement limited to the pelvic lymph nodes—the so-called "cardinal site of metastasis" [13]. This study correlated the incidence and the extent of lymph node involvement with the depth of penetration of the primary bladder tumor, referred to as "an index of curability." These pioneering observations helped form the foundation of the first widely accepted staging system for bladder cancer—the Jewett-Marshall staging system.

---

* Corresponding author.

E-mail address: stein@hsc.usc.edu (J.P. Stein).

0094-0143/05/$ - see front matter © 2005 Elsevier Inc. All rights reserved.
doi:10.1016/j.ucl.2005.01.005

The survival benefits of a pelvic lymphadenectomy in patients with bladder cancer should be first credited to Kerr and Colby [14]. In 1950, they reported long-term survival in two node-positive patients undergoing radical cystectomy with a pelvic lymphadenectomy. In addition, they noted a high incidence of pelvic recurrence following a simple cystectomy. These observations prompted the routine application and inclusion of a lymphadenectomy with wide excision at the time of radical cystectomy, leading to a decrease in pelvic recurrence with improved survival [14]. These experiences helped to direct the contemporary surgical concept of routine lymphadenectomy with wide surgical margins at the time of cystectomy to reduce local recurrences and improve the curability of the disease.

In 1950, Leadbetter elegantly reported his experience, detailing his surgical approach and the boundaries of an extended lymphadenectomy in patients with bladder cancer based on a better understanding of the lymphatic drainage of the bladder and prostate [15]. These boundaries included (1) proximally, the distal aorta; (2) laterally, the genitofemoral nerve; and (3) distally, the recurrent iliac vein (laterally) and the lymph node of Cloquet (medially). Although the specific boundaries or limits of a lymphadenectomy for bladder cancer continue to be debated today, the suggestion even in 1950 was that a more extended lymphadenectomy may be necessary to remove all potential lymph node metastases, including the lymphatics at the level of the distal aorta and vena cava.

Nearly a decade later, Whitmore and Marshall [16] reported their clinical experience in 230 patients with bladder cancer undergoing surgical excision with lymphadenectomy. In this group, 55 patients were found to have D_1 (lymph node positive) disease, with 2 (4%) long-term survivors. Whitmore and Marshall were unaware of any patient with histologic evidence of nodal metastases who survived more than 5 years unless an excision of the primary tumor and the metastases was performed. They concluded that "for patients with only a few pelvic nodal metastases, radical cystectomy has provided some 5-year successful results—the only such of which we are aware." Leadbetter subsequently updated his experience with lymphadenectomy in patients with bladder cancer undergoing cystectomy [17]. This report confirmed the benefit of a lymphadenectomy, with an improved survival in node-positive patients, and was the first to document specifically no

apparent increase in the morbidity and mortality associated with an extended lymph node dissection at the time of radical cystectomy.

In 1982, Skinner [18] reported his pioneering surgical experience with the application of a "meticulous" extended lymph node dissection, with long-term survival in approximately 30% of lymph node–positive patients. Nevertheless, controversy continues regarding the absolute extent (boundaries) of the lymph node dissection in patients undergoing radical cystectomy for bladder cancer. Although some believe that a "standard" dissection (cephalad extent at the level of the common iliac bifurcation) provides adequate staging information, some evidence suggests that a more extended (cephalad extent to include the common iliac vessel and possibly the distal aorta and vena cava) lymphadenectomy is beneficial in patients undergoing cystectomy for bladder cancer, including those with node-positive and node-negative bladder disease.

Lymphatic drainage of the bladder

An anatomic understanding of the lymphatic drainage of the bladder is necessary when considering the specific sites of lymph node metastases and attempting to define the absolute required boundaries of an appropriate lymphadenectomy. The primary contributions to the knowledge of vesical lymphatics have come from European sources and were well summarized by Leadbetter in 1950 [15].

Radical cystectomy series have confirmed that the two most common sites of lymph node involvement are the obturator/hypogastric and external iliac lymph nodes. Smith and Whitmore [19] reported that these sites of nodal metastases were involved in 74% and 65% of cystectomies, respectively. Lymph node metastases were also demonstrated in 19% of cases to the common iliac lymph node packet. This study was one of the first anatomic lymph node mappings in patients undergoing radical cystectomy that suggested the need and importance of an extended lymph node dissection and the removal of all potential lymph node metastases, including those along the common iliac vessels. The need to extend the lymph node dissection to a higher (more cephalad) level remains controversial. Leadbetter initially commented that it was not necessary to describe the aortocaval lymph nodes, because their surgical removal could not be done and should not be part of the cystectomy [15]. In fact, it has been shown that an extended lymphadenectomy, including removal of the lymphatic tissue distal to the inferior mesenteric artery, can be performed safely [3,4]. Furthermore, there is pathologic evidence to suggest that the lymph node region extending from the aortic bifurcation to the level of the inferior mesenteric artery may be a site of nodal metastasis that can be effectively removed surgically [4].

Similar to bladder cancer, prostate cancer preferentially metastasizes to the obturator and external iliac lymph nodes as the first site of lymph node spread [20,21]. In a canine study, the lymphatic drainage of the prostate was carefully evaluated based on the anatomy of the prostate [22]. Lymphatics of the prostate gland were found to drain primarily into the obturator and iliac lymph nodes, but also into the presacral lymph nodes. This finding, coupled with the fact that high-grade invasive bladder cancer can involve the prostate [23], and the knowledge that mapping studies have documented presacral lymph node metastases [4,8] underscore the importance of removing the presacral lymph nodes during lymphadenectomy for bladder cancer.

Recently, the specific distribution of nodal metastases was prospectively evaluated in a multi-center study in which an extended lymphadenectomy was performed in all patients with bladder cancer [4]. This mapping study demonstrated that positive lymph nodes were found most commonly in the obturator spaces and adjacent to the iliac vessels. Interestingly, 16% of lymph node metastases also included nodes above the aortic bifurcation, whereas 8% of lymph node metastases involved the presacral region. Among patients with nodal metastases located within the limits of a standard dissection (below the bifurcation of the common iliacs), a significant proportion of patients also had nodal involvement at the level of the common iliac vessels and above the aortic bifurcation, that is, 57% and 31%, respectively. If the dissection been limited to the obturator spaces, 74% of all positive lymph nodes would have been left behind, and nearly 7% of the patients in this cohort would have been misclassified as node negative [4]. The importance of an extended lymphadenectomy was also corroborated in a study in which 33% of patients with unexpected microscopic nodal involvement at the time of cystectomy had lymph node metastases to the common iliac lymph nodes [24].

A stage-specific lymph node metastasis mapping study was recently reported by Vazina and

colleagues [8]. A total of 176 patients underwent an extended lymphadenectomy with radical cystectomy; 43 patients (24.4%) had pathologic lymph node involvement. Although the most common sites of nodal metastases were the external iliac and hypogastric/obturator regions, 5.1% of patients had presacral nodal involvement, and 9% had disease above the common iliac bifurcation. Importantly, 33% of patients with involvement of the common iliac lymph nodes also had involvement of the presacral region, supporting the importance of removing these nodes as well. Interestingly, a "skip metastasis" occurred in one patient with positive lymph nodes at or above the common iliac bifurcation without involvement of the more distal pelvic lymphatics [8]. Collectively, these studies support the application of an extended lymphadenectomy with a cephalad extent of dissection that includes the distal para-aortic and paracaval lymph nodes, as well as removal of the presacral nodal packet.

The need for a bilateral lymph node dissection has also been questioned, particularly in patients with a unilateral bladder tumor [25,26]. In the mapping study by Leissner et al, bilateral lymph node metastases were commonly seen even if the primary cancer was limited to the right or left hemisphere of the bladder wall [4]. Mills and associates [27] evaluated lymph node metastases in 83 patients with bladder cancer following radical cystectomy and found that 41% of patients with a unilateral bladder tumor had contralateral nodal involvement. In a mapping study of 200 patients undergoing an extended lymphadenectomy, 24% of patients were found to have node-positive disease, and 39% of these cases had bilateral involvement [28]. These data suggest that a bilateral lymphadenectomy is important to remove all potential sites for nodal metastases at the time of cystectomy.

Incidence of bladder cancer with lymph node metastasis at autopsy

The incidence of lymph node–positive disease in autopsy studies suggests that lymph node involvement may be the sole site of metastases in 30% to 40% of patients with bladder cancer. In 1931, Cunningham [29] collected data on 411 cases of bladder cancer that came to autopsy evaluation. Of these, 132 were from the Mayo Clinic, with 17% of the cases demonstrating regional lymph node involvement. Colston and Leadbetter [30] subsequently reported on 98 cases of carcinoma of the bladder coming to autopsy. Metastases were found in 56% of cases, whereas 25% demonstrated only pelvic or retroperitoneal lymph node involvement—a similar incidence documented in radical cystectomy series.

Jewett studied the incidence of lymph node involvement in autopsy cases and was the first to correlate the depth of tumor invasion of the primary bladder tumor to the incidence of lymph node metastases [13]. In this study of 107 autopsies, lymph node involvement was seen in three cases in group A (mucosal infiltration only), in 1 of 15 cases (7%) in group B (extension into the muscular layer), and in 52 of the 89 cases (58%) in group C (extension into the perivesical tissues). Jewett's early observation correlating lymph node metastases with the depth of penetration of the primary tumor has subsequently been confirmed in several large clinical studies of patients undergoing radical cystectomy [3–6,8].

It is reasonable to assume that the incidence of nodal metastases in radical cystectomy patients should be lower than in autopsy studies, because patients considered unresectable or inoperable are generally excluded from analysis. Nevertheless, autopsy studies suggest that (1) a significant number of patients with bladder cancer will have regional lymph node metastases only, (2) these lymph nodes can be removed with an appropriate lymphadenectomy, and (3) the frequency of lymph node tumor metastases correlates to the degree or depth of invasion of the primary bladder tumor.

Incidence of bladder cancer with lymph node metastasis following radical cystectomy

The incidence of lymph node metastases in patients undergoing radical cystectomy is approximately 26% (Table 1) [3–6,8,9]. In the 2815 patients undergoing radical cystectomy with lymphadenectomy in the referenced series, 723 patients (26%) were found to have lymph node metastases. Furthermore, in support of Jewett's early observation, the correlation between the depth of invasion of the primary tumor and the incidence of lymph node metastases is evident (see Table 1).

Surgical boundaries of the lymphadenectomy

An extended lymphadenectomy must include all lymph nodes in the boundaries of the aortic bifurcation and common iliac vessels (proximally),

Table 1
Incidence of lymph node metastasis following radical cystectomy in contemporary series: correlation to primary bladder tumor

Study	Period (years)	Total number of patients	Number (%) with lymph node metastasis	Bladder tumor stage[a], number (%) p0, pis, pa, p1	p2a	p2b	p3	p4
Poulsen et al [5]	1990–1997	191	50 (26%)	2 (3%)	4 (18%)	7 (25%)	33 (51%)	4 (44%)
Vieweg et al[b] [6]	1980–1990	686	193 (28%)	10 (10%)	12 (9%)	22 (23%)	97 (43%)	52 (41%)
Leissner et al[c] [4]	1999–2002	290	81 (28%)	1 (2%)	5 (13%)	12 (22%)	53 (44%)	10 (50%)
Stein et al [3]	1971–1997	1054	246 (24%)	19 (5%)	21 (18%)	35 (27%)	113 (45%)	58 (43%)
Vazina et al[d] [8]	1992–2002	176	43 (24%)	1 (4%)	10 (16%)		20 (40%)	12 (50%)
Abdel-Latif et al[e] [9]	1997–1999	418	110 (26%)	3 (4%)	4 (7%)	29 (25%)	59 (48%)	15 (65%)
		2815	723 (26%)					

[a] TNM staging system, 1997 American Joint Committee on Cancer.
[b] Six patients with carcinoma in situ of prostatic ducts with lymph node–positive disease classified as pis.
[c] Multicentered trial.
[d] p2a and p2b combined.
[e] Includes squamous cell, adenocarcinoma, and TCC of the bladder.

the genitofemoral nerve (laterally), the circumflex iliac vein and lymph node of Cloquet (distally), the hypogastric vessels (posteriorly) including the obturator fossa, presciatic nodes bilaterally, and the presacral lymph nodes. An extended dissection may also reach superiorly to the level of the inferior mesenteric artery. A so-called "standard" lymphadenectomy is more limited, with the cephalad extent generally beginning at the level of the common iliac bifurcation. The lateral and distal limits are similar to the extended dissection.

Factors influencing the number of lymph nodes evaluated or retrieved

Lymphadenectomy in patients undergoing radical cystectomy is a diagnostic tool that provides staging and possibly therapeutic benefits as well. The number of lymph nodes assessed pathologically depends on several factors, including (1) the boundaries of the lymph node dissection (extended versus standard or even more limited), (2) the pathologist's diligence in searching and preparing the lymph nodes for histopathologic evaluation, and (3) how the specimen is actually submitted for pathologic evaluation. These factors may collectively contribute to determining the actual number of lymph nodes retrieved and the exact incidence and extent of lymph node tumor involvement.

Diligent pathologic evaluation is essential in the identification of the total number of nodes removed and the extent of nodal metastases. In general, most lymph nodes are identified visually and by palpation, without the need of clearing techniques or solvents. Using this technique in a large group of 244 patients with lymph node–positive disease undergoing an en bloc radical cystectomy and extended lymphadenectomy, a median number of 30 lymph nodes were removed and evaluated [31]. It has recently been suggested that to facilitate nodal evaluation, separate nodal packets should be submitted intraoperatively by the surgeon [32]. By simply converting from an en bloc technique to submission of six separate lymph node packets (maintaining the limits of dissection), the mean number of lymph nodes removed is increased by more than threefold [32]. The authors have adopted a similar approach at their center with the submission of 12 individual lymph node packets. This modification has significantly increased the median number of lymph nodes removed and evaluated from 30 to 56, with specific tumor location (Stein JP, MD, 2004, unpublished data).

The absolute limits of the lymph node dissection may be the most important factor and may have the greatest impact on the number of lymph nodes removed during cystectomy. In two large cystectomy series in which an extended lymphadenectomy was performed, the median number of lymph nodes removed ranged from 30 to 43 [4,31]. Extending the boundaries of the lymph node dissection, Poulsen et al reported an increase in the average number of lymph nodes removed from 14 in a standard dissection to 25 when the dissection was carried up to the bifurcation of the aorta [5]. Bochner et al [32] confirmed these findings, reporting a significantly greater number of nodes removed with an extended dissection when compared with a more standard dissection, that is, 36.5 versus 8.5, respectively.

Clearly, the influence of the surgeon and pathologist is an important factor in determining the lymph node count and involvement of tumor. Although the exact number of nodes that should be removed at the time of cystectomy is unknown, extending the limits of the dissection and submitting the lymph nodes in packets increases the number of lymph nodes retrieved and evaluated. Fat-clearing immunohistochemical and molecular techniques may increase the nodal counts, but these specialized methods are more expensive, time consuming, and may not necessarily provide additional prognostic information, particularly if an extended lymphadenectomy is performed. In fact, a recent report evaluated various factors that contributed to the variability in the number of lymph nodes removed at cystectomy; only the extent of the lymph node dissection was found to influence significantly the nodal yield [24].

Required number of lymph nodes that must be removed

Many factors may influence the surgical approach and extent of lymphadenectomy in patients with bladder cancer. Patient age, associated comorbidities, and the extent of disease may all have a role in the decision process. In addition, the comfort and experience of the surgeon is important. In patients with prostate cancer, experienced urologic oncologists performing radical prostatectomy in high-volume centers tend to achieve better outcomes when compared with surgeons performing fewer cases in low-volume institutions [33]. This observation may also apply to radical cystectomy. Interestingly, in a recent analysis of the Surveillance, Epidemiology, and

End Results (SEER) Program cancer registry, only 40% of patients who underwent cystectomy for bladder cancer had a lymph node dissection, and in half of all eligible patients, urologists elected not to perform a cystectomy at all [34]. It is apparent that the surgical management of bladder cancer in the United States varies tremendously. Despite a growing body of evidence suggesting that an aggressive surgical approach with an appropriate lymphadenectomy may benefit patients, this is not always performed.

Suggested guidelines for the surgical approach and clinical outcomes of patients with TCC undergoing cystectomy have been proposed. A multicentered report from the Bladder Cancer Collaborative Group evaluated and suggested surgical standards for radical cystectomy [35]. Sixteen experienced surgeons from four academic institutions contributed 1091 cystectomy patients over a 3-year period. It was concluded that at least 10 yearly cystectomies are required to maintain proficiency. At least 10 to 14 lymph nodes should be retrieved, with a margin-positive rate of fewer than 10% of all cases (less than 15% for bulky tumors and less than 20% for salvage cases) performed. A complete/standard lymphadenectomy correlated with fewer positive margins and increased node counts in patients with positive and negative nodal disease [35]. This finding also argues for a more extensive lymphadenectomy in patients undergoing radical cystectomy for bladder cancer.

Morbidity and mortality of lymphadenectomy

Understanding that a lymph node dissection is important in the management of patients undergoing radical cystectomy for bladder cancer, coupled with the fact that a more extensive lymphadenectomy may provide more accurate pathologic staging and survival benefits, one must carefully evaluate the risks associated with an extended lymph node dissection. This issue is particularly important in patients with bladder cancer who tend to be elderly with associated comorbidities.

In the authors' series of 1054 patients uniformly undergoing an extended lymphadenectomy, the reported perioperative mortality rate was 3%, with an early complication rate of 28% [3]. There were no perioperative deaths or early complications related directly to the lymph node dissection. Furthermore, in the subgroup analysis of patients with lymph node–positive disease, the operative

mortality rate was 1%, with an early complication rate of 27% [31]. No differences were noted when comparing this pathologic group with patients with organ-confined and extravesical tumors without lymph node tumor metastases. These findings have been confirmed recently in a study that questioned whether an extended lymphadenectomy would increase morbidity in patients undergoing radical cystectomy [36]. Forty-six patients undergoing an extended lymphadenectomy (cephalad dissection at the level of the inferior mesenteric artery) were compared with 46 patients undergoing a minimal dissection (cephalad extent at the region of the common iliac artery bifurcation). Patients were well matched with regard to associated comorbidities and American Society of Anesthesiologists grade. Overall, 30% of patients were found to have lymph node metastases. Although the extended lymphadenectomy increased the operative duration by approximately 60 minutes, there was no significant difference in perioperative mortality, early complications, or the need for blood transfusions between the two groups. It was concluded that, despite prolonging the operation, an extended lymphadenectomy did not result in an increased complication rate during or after (within 30 days following) surgery [36].

In a retrospective analysis, the outcomes of an extended lymph node dissection (cephalad limits at the level of the aortic bifurcation) were compared with those of a more limited pelvic lymph node dissection bounded proximally by the bifurcation of the common iliac vessels [5]. The lateral, distal, and posterior dissections were similar. As expected, the median number of lymph nodes removed was significantly higher in the extended group when compared with the limited group. There was no difference in mortality. Lymphocele formation occurred in two (1.6%) patients in the extended group and one (1.5%) patient in the limited group [5]. Similar findings were seen in patients undergoing cystectomy and an extended node dissection. In 447 patients, lymphoceles and lymphedema were observed in 2% of patients with less than 16 lymph nodes removed and in 1% of patients with 16 or more lymph nodes removed [7]. Collectively, these studies suggest the morbidity associated with an extended lymphadenectomy is low and comparable with that in a more limited node dissection.

A recent multicenter study prospectively evaluated the role of an extended lymphadenectomy in 290 patients undergoing cystectomy for bladder cancer [4]. Although the extended lymph node dissection required 60 minutes longer to perform, during the immediate postoperative period, none of the participating centers observed any significant adverse effects related to the extended lymphadenectomy. In some cases, there was increased postoperative lymphatic drainage; however, all drains were safely removed 3 to 10 days following the operation [4].

Even in experienced hands, an extended lymphadenectomy may take 30 to 60 minutes longer than a more limited dissection. The surgeon should be committed to performing a complete and meticulous lymphadenectomy. Experience in lymph node dissection along large vessels is helpful. The surgeon should feel comfortable with the basic premises of vascular surgery and should have a sound understanding of the regional anatomy. If properly performed, an extended lymph node dissection sets up the remaining portion of the operation, which can then be performed safely with proper vascular control, and reduces the potential for significant blood loss. Furthermore, this surgical approach helps reduce the incidence of positive surgical margins [35].

Prognostic factors in patients with lymph node metastases following radical cystectomy

To provide risk stratification and to direct the need for adjuvant treatment therapies, various prognostic factors have been identified in patients with lymph node metastases following radical cystectomy. Traditional risk factors stratifying patients with lymph node metastases include the extent of the primary bladder tumor (p stage) and the total number of lymph nodes involved with tumor (tumor burden). There is also evidence to suggest that the survival in these patients is affected by the extent of the lymphadenectomy, reflected by the number of lymph nodes removed. The concept of lymph node density has also been found to provide significant prognostic information in patients with lymph node–positive disease following radical cystectomy.

Number of lymph nodes involved (tumor burden)

The number of positive lymph nodes, or the number of lymph nodes involved with tumor (tumor burden), is an important prognostic factor in patients with bladder cancer following radical cystectomy [3,7,9,15,19,27,31,37–43]. As expected, survival and recurrence are inversely related to an increasing tumor burden. Smith and Whitmore initially reported on 134 patients with lymph node

metastases following radical cystectomy and found that survival directly correlated with the number of lymph nodes involved [19]. Lerner et al reported on 132 patients with nodal metastases and found that patients with five positive lymph nodes or less had a significantly better recurrence-free and overall survival when compared with patients with six or more lymph nodes involved with tumor [37].

Herr and associates examined a cohort of 322 patients undergoing radical cystectomy. Among the 64 (20%) patients with node-positive disease, survival was significantly improved if patients had four or fewer positive lymph nodes when compared with patients who had greater than four positive lymph nodes (37% versus 13%, respectively) [43]. Furthermore, in this node-positive group of patients, if more than 11 lymph nodes were removed (total), an improved survival with better local pelvic control of the tumor was observed. These data underscore the importance of a more extended lymphadenectomy in patients with node-positive bladder cancer. Interestingly, in the study of 258 lymph node–negative patients, survival was also directly proportional to the number of lymph nodes removed. The researchers appropriately commented that identifying a greater number of lymph nodes might reflect a more complete radical cystectomy and lymphadenectomy in lymph node–positive and negative patients. These findings were subsequently supported in a larger group of 148 node-positive patients by the same researcher [44].

Several other studies have supported the correlation between the number of lymph node metastases and survival in patients following radical cystectomy. In the largest reported series of 244 lymph node–positive patients with long-term follow-up (median, 10 years), the number of lymph nodes involved with tumor was a significant and independent prognostic factor regarding survival [31]. Patients with eight or fewer positive lymph nodes demonstrated significantly higher survival when compared with patients with more than eight positive lymph nodes. The 5- and 10-year recurrence-free survival rates for patients with eight or less positive lymph nodes were 41% and 40%, respectively, compared with a 10% recurrence-free survival at 10-years when more than eight lymph nodes were involved with tumor [31].

Extent of the primary bladder tumor (p stage)

The prognosis of patients with node-positive disease following radical cystectomy is strongly associated with the pathologic stage of the primary bladder tumor (p stage) [3,9,25,31,37,38,42]. Vieweg et al demonstrated that survival was significantly related to the stage of the primary tumor in 193 patients with node-positive disease following cystectomy [38]. In their series, patients with organ-confined (p0-p3a) node-positive disease had a 58% probability of surviving 5 years compared with a 22% 5-year survival rate for patients with extravesical lymph node–positive disease. The authors' group reported that the recurrence-free and overall survival in 244 patients with lymph node–positive disease was significantly related to the pathologic subgroup (organ-confined versus extravesical) of the primary bladder tumor [31]. Patients with organ-confined, lymph node–positive tumors demonstrated a 5- and 10-year recurrence-free survival of 46% and 44%, respectively. These survival rates were significantly better than the 30% 5- and 10-year rates for patients with extravesical lymph node–positive disease. Furthermore, in a multivariate analysis, the extent of the primary bladder tumor remained a significant and independent prognostic factor in patients with lymph node–positive tumors [38]. Similar findings were reported in the study by the Mansoura group. The primary bladder tumor stage significantly influenced the incidence and survival in patients with node-positive disease following radical cystectomy [9].

Number of lymph nodes removed (extent of lymphadenectomy)

The number of lymph nodes removed at the time of cystectomy is related to the extent or completeness of the lymph node dissection performed. As mentioned previously, Poulsen et al demonstrated that extending the limits of the node dissection from the bifurcation of the common iliac vessels up to the level of the aortic bifurcation increased the median number of lymph nodes removed from 14 to 25 [5]. Although the absolute limits or extent of the lymph node dissection has not been precisely defined, a growing body of data suggests that a minimum number of lymph nodes should be removed and evaluated pathologically during radical cystectomy [7,31,34,35,39,41,43,44].

The extent of the lymphadenectomy (number of lymph nodes removed) seems to have prognostic significance in lymph node–positive and lymph node–negative patients with bladder cancer following radical cystectomy. Herr reported on 667 patients undergoing radical cystectomy: 489

(77%) node-negative patients and 148 (23%) node-positive patients [43]. Survival for lymph node–negative and positive patients was improved, with a reduced local recurrence rate, when a greater number of lymph nodes were removed. Leissner et al evaluated 447 patients who underwent radical cystectomy and also found a significantly improved survival if a greater number of lymph nodes were removed [7]. This finding was true for patients without lymph node metastases and for patients with five positive lymph nodes or less. If more than 16 lymph nodes were removed, the 5-year recurrence-free survival rate increased from 63% to 85% in organ-confined tumors, from 40% to 55% in pT3 tumors, and from 25% to 53% in patients with at most five lymph node metastases. Furthermore, if at least 20 lymph nodes were removed, approximately 80% of lymph node–positive patients would be identified, suggesting that this would be a reasonable number of lymph nodes to be removed and evaluated at cystectomy [7].

Similarly, Poulsen and associates demonstrated that extending the limits of the pelvic lymph node dissection provided a benefit in a subset of patients with organ-confined, lymph node–negative bladder tumors [5]. The 5-year recurrence-free survival with organ-confined, node-negative tumors was 85% with an extended dissection compared with 64% with similar pathology undergoing a more limited dissection. Furthermore, an extended dissection reduced the pelvic and distant metastases rate in these patients [5]. Additional confirmation comes from an analysis of more than 20,000 patients with bladder cancer (1923 patients undergoing cystectomy) included in the SEER cancer registry [34]. In this large cohort, the risk of death was significantly higher in patients with less than four lymph nodes removed at cystectomy, independent of stage and lymph node–positive disease. The most important survival factor in patients undergoing cystectomy, effectively controlling for age, tumor stage, histology, chemotherapy, and radiotherapy, was the removal of 10 to 14 lymph nodes at the time of surgery [34].

It is speculated that an extended lymph node dissection (in lymph node–positive and negative patients) may remove undetected lymph node micrometastases, improving survival in patients undergoing cystectomy. Despite these data suggesting that a greater number of lymph nodes removed at the time of cystectomy is beneficial for all patients, and that an extended lymph node dissection will remove a greater number of lymph nodes, no uniform consensus exists regarding the limits or absolute boundary of the lymph node dissection, or the minimum number of lymph nodes that should be removed.

Lymph node density (number of lymph nodes involved/number of lymph nodes removed)

Both the extent of the lymphadenectomy and lymph node tumor burden are known to be important risk factors in patients undergoing radical cystectomy. To account for the number of lymph nodes removed (extent of the lymph node dissection) and the total number of lymph nodes involved (tumor burden), the concept of lymph node density for patients with node-positive bladder cancer has been suggested [31]. Lymph node density is defined as the number of lymph nodes involved with tumor divided by the total number of lymph nodes removed. If tumor burden and the extent of the lymphadenectomy are important variables in patients with node-positive bladder cancer, it is logical that lymph node density should also be prognostic. In the authors' group of 244 lymph node–positive patients, lymph node density was found to be a significant and independent prognostic factor. Patients with a lymph node density of 20% or less demonstrated a 43% 10-year recurrence-free survival rate compared with a 17% survival rate at 10 years when the lymph node density was greater than 20% [31].

Herr recently published his findings regarding this concept of lymph node density described as ratio-based lymph node staging [39]. In 162 patients with lymph node–positive disease, this ratio system better defined the surgical outcomes. The 5-year survival rate in patients with node-positive disease and a lymph node density of less than 20% was 64%, significantly higher than the 8% 5-year survival for the same pathologic group of patients with a lymph node density greater than 20% [39]. Similarly, the proportion of positive lymph nodes to excised lymph nodes (lymph node density) for metastatic bladder cancer correlated with the risk of death from bladder cancer in the SEER registry of patients undergoing radical cystectomy [34].

The concept of lymph node density collectively accounts for lymph node burden and the extent of lymph node dissection, both of which clearly have prognostic significance. Lymph node density better stratifies lymph node–positive patients into various risk groups, which may be useful in future staging systems. Furthermore, future adjuvant therapies and clinical trials should consider applying this concept, because it may help reduce the surgical bias and extent of the lymphadenectomy, both of which are not standardized.

Summary

Radical cystectomy with bilateral pelvic iliac lymphadenectomy is a standard treatment for high-grade, invasive bladder cancer. Cystectomy arguably provides the best survival outcomes and the lowest local recurrence rates. Although the extent or absolute limits of the lymph node dissection are unknown and remain to be better defined, an ever-growing body of data supports a more extended lymphadenectomy at the time of cystectomy in all patients who are appropriate surgical candidates. An extended lymph node dissection should include the distal para-aortic and paracaval lymph nodes as well as the presacral nodes, known anatomic sites of lymph node drainage from the bladder and potential sites of lymph node metastases in patients with bladder cancer. An extended dissection may provide a survival advantage in patients with node-positive and node-negative tumors without significantly increasing the morbidity or mortality of the surgery. The extent of the primary bladder tumor (p stage), the number of lymph nodes removed, and the lymph node tumor burden are important prognostic variables in patients undergoing cystectomy with pathologic evidence of lymph node metastases. Lymph node density may become an even more useful prognostic variable in these high-risk, node-positive patients with bladder cancer. This concept simultaneously incorporates the lymph node tumor burden (number of lymph nodes involved) and the number of lymph nodes removed (extent of the lymphadenectomy), improving the stratification of lymph node–positive patients following radical cystectomy. This notion may also be useful in future staging systems. Adjuvant therapies and clinical trials should consider applying these concepts, because they may help reduce bias and incorporate the extent of the lymphadenectomy, which currently is not standardized.

References

[1] Jemal A, Tiwari RC, Murray T, et al. Cancer statistics, 2004. CA Cancer J Clin 2004;54:8–29.

[2] Stein JP. Indications for early cystectomy. Urology 2003;62:591–5.

[3] Stein JP, Lieskovsky G, Cote R, et al. Radical cystectomy in the treatment of invasive bladder cancer: long-term results in 1054 patients. J Clin Oncol 2001; 19:666–75.

[4] Leissner J, Ghoneim MA, Abol-Enein H, et al. Extended radical lymphadenectomy in patients with urothelial bladder cancer: results of a prospective multicenter study. J Urol 2004;171:139–44.

[5] Poulsen AL, Horn T, Steven K. Radical cystectomy: extending limits of pelvic lymph node dissection improves survival for patients with bladder cancer confined to the bladder wall. J Urol 1998;160: 2015–20.

[6] Vieweg J, Gschwend JE, Herr HW, et al. The impact of primary stage on survival in patients with lymph node positive bladder cancer. J Urol 1999; 161:72–6.

[7] Leissner J, Hohenfellner R, Thuroff JW, et al. Lymphadenectomy in patients with transitional cell carcinoma of the urinary bladder; significance for staging and prognosis. BJU Int 2000;85:817–23.

[8] Vazina A, Dugi D, Shariat SF, et al. Stage specific lymph node metastasis mapping in radical cystectomy specimens. J Urol 2004;171:1830–4.

[9] Abdel-Latif M, Abol-Enein H, El-Baz M, et al. Nodal involvement in bladder cancer cases treated with radical cystectomy: incidence and prognosis. J Urol 2004;172:85–9.

[10] Barth PJ, Gerharz EW, Ramaswamy A, et al. The influence of lymph node counts on the detection of pelvic lymph node metastasis in prostate cancer. Pathol Res Pract 1999;195:633–6.

[11] Terrone C, Guercio S, DeLuca S, et al. The number of lymph nodes examined and staging accuracy in renal cell carcinoma. BJU Int 2003;91:37–40.

[12] Colston JA, Leadbetter WF. Infiltrating carcinoma of the bladder. J Urol 1936;36:669–89.

[13] Jewett HJ, Strong GH. Infiltrating carcinoma of the bladder: relation of depth of penetration of the bladder wall to incidence of local extension and metastases. J Urol 1946;55:366–72.

[14] Kerr WS, Colby FH. Pelvic lymph node dissection and total cystectomy in the treatment of carcinoma of the bladder. J Urol 1950;63:842–51.

[15] Leadbetter WF, Cooper JF. Regional gland dissection for carcinoma of the bladder: a technique of one-stage cystectomy, gland dissection and bilateral ureteroenterostomy. J Urol 1950;63:242–60.

[16] Whitmore WF, Marshall VF. Radical total cystectomy for cancer of the bladder: 230 consecutive cases five years later. J Urol 1962;87:853–68.

[17] Dretler SP, Ragsdale BD, Leadbetter WF. The value of pelvic lymphadenectomy in the surgical treatment of bladder cancer. J Urol 1973;109:414–6.

[18] Skinner DG. Management of invasive bladder cancer: a meticulous pelvic node dissection can make a difference. J Urol 1982;128:34–6.

[19] Smith JA, Whitmore WF Jr. Regional lymph node metastasis from bladder cancer. J Urol 1981;126: 591–3.

[20] Donohue RE, Pfister RR, Weigel JW, et al. Pelvic lymphadenectomy in stage A prostatic cancer. Urology 1977;9:273–5.

[21] Wilson CS, Dahl DS, Middleton RG. Pelvic lymphadenectomy for staging of apparently localized prostate cancer. J Urol 1977;117:197–8.

[22] Suzuki T, Kurokawa K, Yamanaks H, et al. Lymphatic drainage of the prostate gland in canines. Prostate 1992;21:279–86.

[23] Esrig D, Freeman JA, Stein JP, et al. Transitional cell carcinoma involving the prostate with a proposed staging classification for stromal invasion. J Urol 1996;156:1071–6.

[24] Bochner BH, Cho C, Herr HW, et al. Prospective packaged lymph node dissections with radical cystectomy: evaluation of node count variability and node mapping. J Urol 2004;172:1286–90.

[25] Wishnow KI, Johnson DE, Ro JY, et al. Incidence, extent and location of unsuspected pelvic lymph node metastasis in patients undergoing radical cystectomy for bladder cancer. J Urol 1987;137:408–10.

[26] Ravery V, Chopin DK, Abbou CC. Anatomie chirurgicale du drainage lymphatique de la vessie. Ann Urol 1993;27:9.

[27] Mills RD, Turner WH, Fleischmann R, et al. Pelvic lymph node metastasis from bladder cancer: outcome in 83 patients after radical cystectomy and pelvic lymphadenectomy. J Urol 2001;166:19–23.

[28] Abol-Enein H, El-Baz M, Abd El-Hameed MA, et al. Lymph node involvement in patients with bladder cancer treated with radical cystectomy: a pathoanatomical study—a single center experience. J Urol 2004;172:1818–21.

[29] Cunningham JH. Tumors of the bladder. J Urol 1931;25:559–87.

[30] Colston JAC, Leadbetter WF. Infiltrating carcinoma of the bladder. J Urol 1936;36:669–89.

[31] Stein JP, Cai J, Groshen S, et al. Risk factors for patients with pelvic lymph node metastases following radical cystectomy with en bloc pelvic lymphadenectomy: the concept of lymph node density. J Urol 2003;170:35–41.

[32] Bochner BH, Herr HW, Reuter VE. Impact of separate versus en bloc pelvic lymph node dissection on the number of lymph nodes retrieved in cystectomy specimens. J Urol 2001;166:2295–6.

[33] Eastham JA, Kattan MW, Riedel E, et al. Variations among individual surgeons in the rate of positive surgical margins in radical prostatectomy specimens. J Urol 2003;170:2292–5.

[34] Konety BR, Joslyn SA, O'Donnell MA. Extent of pelvic lymphadenectomy and its impact on outcome in patients diagnosed with bladder cancer: analysis of data from the surveillance, epidemiology and end results program data base. J Urol 2003;169: 945–50.

[35] Herr H, Lee C, Chang S, et al, for the Bladder Cancer Collaborative Group. Standardization of radical cystectomy and pelvic lymph node dissection for bladder cancer: a collaborative group report. J Urol 2004;171:1823–8.

[36] Brossner C, Pycha A, Toth A, et al. Does extended lymphadenectomy increase the morbidity of radical cystectomy? BJU Int 2004;93:64–6.

[37] Lerner SP, Skinner DG, Lieskovsky G, et al. The rationale for en bloc pelvic lymph node dissection for bladder cancer patients with nodal metastases: long-term results. J Urol 1993;149:758–64.

[38] Viewig J, Gschwend JE, Herr HW, et al. Pelvic lymph node dissection can be curative in patients with node positive bladder cancer. J Urol 1999;161:449–54.

[39] Herr HW. Superiority of ratio based lymph node staging for bladder cancer. J Urol 2003;169:943–5.

[40] Frank I, Cheville JC, Blute ML, et al. Transitional cell carcinoma of the urinary bladder with regional lymph node involvement treated by cystectomy. Cancer 2003;97:2425–31.

[41] Knap MM, Lundbeck F, Overgaard J. The role of pelvic lymph node dissection as a predictive and prognostic factor in bladder cancer. Eur J Cancer 2003;39:604–13.

[42] Vieweg J, Whitmore WF Jr, Herr HW, et al. The role of pelvic lymphadenectomy and radical cystectomy for lymph node positive bladder cancer. Cancer 1994;73:3020–8.

[43] Herr HW, Bochner BH, Dalbagni G, et al. Impact of the number of lymph nodes retrieved on outcome in patients with muscle invasive bladder cancer. J Urol 2002;167:1295–8.

[44] Herr HW. Extent of surgery and pathology evaluation has an impact on bladder cancer outcomes after radical cystectomy. Urology 2003;61:105–8.

ELSEVIER
SAUNDERS

Urol Clin N Am 32 (2005) 199–206

UROLOGIC
CLINICS
of North America

Contemporary Management of the Urethra in Patients After Radical Cystectomy for Bladder Cancer

Peter E. Clark, MD*, M. Craig Hall, MD

*Department of Urology, Wake Forest University Health Sciences,
Medical Center Boulevard, Winston-Salem, NC 27104, USA*

An estimated 60,240 new cases of bladder cancer were expected to be diagnosed in 2004. Of these, approximately 30% to 40% were expected to present with or ultimately develop muscle invasive disease [1]. In the United States, the most accepted management of patients with muscle invasive disease is radical cystectomy with bilateral pelvic lymph node dissection [2]. With removal of the bladder, management of the urethra becomes an important consideration. Several decades ago, the prognosis of patients with symptomatic recurrence of transitional cell carcinoma (TCC) in the urethra was poor [3,4]; therefore, some early investigators advocated routine en bloc removal of the urethra in men and women at the time of cystectomy [4]. This recommendation was based on the rationale that the retained "dry" urethra was of no significant value to the patient and served only as a source of potential morbidity and mortality, analogous to the distal ureter in patients with upper tract TCC. The major argument against routine en bloc urethral resection at the time of cystectomy was based primarily on reports demonstrating increased postoperative morbidity in these men [5–7]. Currently, owing to the pioneering work of Camey and the growing acceptance of orthotopic urinary diversion, management of the retained urethra after radical cystectomy has taken on new importance [8]. This review discusses urethral TCC after radical cystectomy, with particular emphasis on its incidence, risk factors for recurrence, diagnosis, screening tests, and the treatment and outcome among these patients.

Urethral involvement by TCC after radical cystectomy could arguably be due to synchronous or metachronous disease. The urethral involvement may occur owing to unrecognized TCC in the urethra at the time of cystectomy, growth of TCC from a positive margin, recurrence owing to tumor spillage or implantation, or de novo TCC that arises owing to the "field change" throughout the urothelium of patients with TCC. Although it is difficult to assign with certainty each episode of urethral "recurrence" after cystectomy to one of these categories, it is generally believed that most urethral TCC after cystectomy is caused by de novo metachronous development of urethral disease analogous to the development of upper tract TCC [9]. Nevertheless, because of the inherent uncertainty in determining whether urethral involvement by TCC after cystectomy is truly a recurrence, the terms *urethral TCC* and *urethral recurrence* are used interchangeably throughout the remainder of this article.

Rate of urethral transitional cell carcinoma in men

The reported incidence of urethral TCC after radical cystectomy has ranged from 0% to 18% across several series [3,8,10–30]. An early attempt to pool the data from series before 1994 estimated the overall incidence rate to be 10.1% [9]. More recently, a meta-analysis pooling the results from that study along with five additional series concluded that the overall incidence after cystectomy was 8.1% [31]. In one of the largest contemporary cystectomy series from the University of Southern California, the rate was 7.9% [26]. The overall rate of urethral TCC is approximately 8% to 10% across all patients.

* Corresponding author.
E-mail address: peclark@wfubmc.edu (P.E. Clark).

The median time to recurrence across series has ranged from 1.5 to 2.2 years, with most recurrences occurring before 5 years [10,11,19,26,32–34]. Some cases of urethral TCC are diagnosed up to 20 years after radical cystectomy [4,26,32]; therefore, it is critical that the retained urethra, whether "dry" or still functionally associated with an orthotopic diversion, be monitored for the remaining lifetime of the patient.

Risk factors in men

A variety of cancer characteristics have been associated with the incidence of urethral TCC after radical cystectomy in men. These factors include multifocal disease [10,11,13,18,20,22,25, 35–38], the presence of carcinoma in situ (CIS) [10,20,37,39], upper tract TCC [4,11,20,23,37], involvement of the bladder neck with tumor [10,11,20,25], and involvement of the prostatic urethra [10–12,20,22,39,40]. Data for the majority of these risk factors are contradictory and have been discussed extensively in previous reviews [9,41,42]. As noted previously, the presence of CIS has been associated with urethral TCC in several series. Other series have refuted this claim and reported rates of urethral TCC for patients with pathologic CIS of the bladder ranging from 4.5% to 5% [11,12], comparable with the overall rate of 8% to 10% among unselected patients.

Across studies, the most consistent risk factor for urethral TCC after radical cystectomy in men is prostatic involvement [10–12,20,22,39,40]. Ashworth first reported this association when examining seven patients with urethral TCC, five of whom (71%) had a history of prostatic TCC [25]. This risk seems to be directly proportional to the degree to which the prostate is involved. A study by Hardeman and Soloway reviewed their experience with 30 patients who had TCC of the prostate; 11 (37%) urethral recurrences were reported overall [12]. There were no recurrences among the patients with TCC confined to the mucosa, 25% in patients with ductal involvement, and 67% in patients with stromal invasion. Similarly, a report by Levinson et al demonstrated a strong association between prostatic TCC and urethral recurrence after radical cystectomy [11]. Of the six urethral recurrences reviewed, 67% had a history of prostatic TCC. Again, this rate was directly proportional to the depth of involvement. There were no recurrences among patients with only mucosal involvement, whereas the rates for

those with ductal involvement or stromal invasion were 10% and 30%, respectively. In another study of 436 radical cystectomy patients, the 5-year probability of urethral recurrence was 6% for patients without prostatic TCC involvement compared with 15% for patients with superficial involvement and 21% for those with stromal invasion of the prostate ($P = .0002$) [26]. Taken together, the literature demonstrates that the most important risk factor for urethral recurrence is prostatic stromal invasion.

The question has been raised whether men who are candidates for radical cystectomy should undergo routine biopsy of the prostatic urethra before surgery to determine their eligibility for orthotopic diversion. A prospective series of 118 patients by Lebret et al has examined the utility of preoperative prostatic biopsies versus intraoperative frozen section analysis of the prostatic urethral margin at the time of cystectomy in predicting urethral recurrence [27]. They found that intraoperative frozen section was more accurate than any preoperative parameter, including preoperative prostate biopsies, in predicting urethral recurrence. As a result, it is routine practice at the authors' center and many others to base a patient's eligibility for orthotopic diversion, at least with respect to the risk for urethral TCC, on intraoperative frozen section analysis at the time of radical cystectomy. It is imperative that a full discussion take place with the patient before surgery on the preferred option (ie, conduit versus continent cutaneous reservoir) should the frozen section be positive [26,27].

Risk factors in women

It is almost universally accepted that women who are not undergoing orthotopic diversion should undergo en bloc resection of the entire urethra at the time of cystectomy, because this step adds minimal time or morbidity to the operation [31]. The risk of urethral TCC in women has become an issue only since the introduction and popularization of orthotopic diversion among carefully selected women undergoing radical cystectomy in the early 1990s [43–48]. The estimated overall risk of urethral TCC in women at the time of cystectomy is not as well studied as in men. An early report by Ashworth found an incidence of 1.4% among 293 women [25]. In a large series of 356 women undergoing radical cystectomy, the incidence of urethral involvement by TCC on final pathology was 2% overall and only 1% among women without nodal involvement or invasion into adjacent viscera (T2-T3, N0, M0 disease) [49]. Although several factors are associated with the risk of urethral TCC in women at the time of cystectomy, the most consistent association is with TCC of the bladder neck [49–51]. Nevertheless, it remains controversial whether involvement of the bladder neck is an absolute contraindication to orthotopic diversion in women, or whether that distinction can be made by intraoperative frozen section analysis, similar to the approach in men [31,51]. A recent review by Stenzl et al suggested that, given the risk for urethral TCC at the time of cystectomy in women with involvement of the bladder neck, all women should undergo preoperative biopsies of the bladder neck, and women who demonstrate overt tumor or atypia at this location should undergo a total urethrectomy [31,52]. Conversely, a prospective pathologic evaluation of 71 women undergoing radical cystectomy suggested that, although all women with urethral TCC on the final cystectomy pathologic analysis had bladder neck involvement, more than 60% of women with bladder neck involvement had no evidence of urethral TCC [51]. Intraoperative frozen section analysis was performed in 47 of these women. That analysis accurately predicted involvement of the urethra by TCC in every case (2 with and 45 without urethral TCC). It was suggested that a consideration of orthotopic diversion can be made based on frozen section analysis at the time of radical cystectomy, and that, as is true in men, careful preoperative counseling is required in the event the intraoperative analysis is positive for TCC. Although it is generally agreed that a women with overt tumor in the urethra should undergo total urethrectomy at the time of cystectomy, there is no consensus on the appropriate management for women with TCC at the bladder neck.

Interestingly, there are few reported cases of urethral TCC in women after radical cystectomy and orthotopic urinary diversion. A recent review of a large cystectomy database that included 44 women who had undergone cystectomy and orthotopic diversion reported no urethral TCC at last follow-up [32]. The only case report of urethral TCC in a woman after orthotopic diversion was published recently [53]. Given the ever-increasing number of women who are successfully undergoing orthotopic urinary diversion, the rarity of case reports suggests that the incidence of urethral TCC after orthotopic diversion is low. A more accurate estimate of the rate at which urethral TCC occurs in women after radical cystectomy and orthotopic diversion awaits long-term follow-up and study.

Orthotopic diversion and the risk for urethral transitional cell carcinoma

In men, the incidence of urethral TCC after orthotopic diversion may be lower than in men who undergo a cutaneous urinary diversion in whom the urethra is "dry." A carefully analyzed study by Freeman et al [26] compared 174 men who had undergone orthotopic urinary diversion after radical cystectomy with 262 men who had undergone a form of cutaneous urinary diversion. The overall rate of urethral recurrence in this series was 7.9% at a median time of 1.6 years after cystectomy. The 5-year actuarial risk of recurrence was significantly greater for patients undergoing cutaneous urinary diversion (11.1%) when compared with patients undergoing orthotopic diversion (2.9%, $P = .015$). Among patients with prostatic involvement by TCC, the recurrence rate was 5% in those who underwent orthotopic diversion compared with 24% among those who had cutaneous diversion ($P = .05$). There has been speculation as to the possible mechanisms that could account for this observation. Theories include the possible excretion of a protective substance by the ileum, a protective effect of continued exposure to urine, or some systemic effect of undergoing an orthotopic versus cutaneous urinary diversion. To date, the study by Freeman et al is the only report to have directly studied this observation, and these findings await confirmation by other studies.

Monitoring the urethra after cystectomy

It is intuitive that the patient with a retained urethra after cystectomy should be monitored for the possibility of urethral TCC. At a minimum, this follow-up should include annual cytology and full evaluation, including urethroscopy, in patients who experience symptoms related to the urethra. A recent study examined the diagnosis and management of urethral TCC among 47 patients after radical cystectomy [32]. Although most patients in that study were symptomatic, among the 37 patients in whom urethral TCC was detected during long-term follow-up, cytologic screening alone diagnosed 13 of the patients (35%). Among the patients with cytology data available, 94% had a positive cytology. The utility of urinary cytology in this setting has also been reported by Wolinska et al [54]. In that study, among 24 patients with a positive cytology, 21 were found to have a tumor, whereas 3 (12.5%) had a false-positive cytology. These findings suggest that urethral wash or voided cytology is an important part of any surveillance protocol after radical cystectomy for TCC.

Symptomatic patients with urethral TCC usually present with bloody urethral discharge or gross hematuria [4,32]. Nevertheless, in the previously mentioned study of a large cohort of patients with urethral TCC after cystectomy, 4 of the 14 patients with an orthotopic neobladder in whom a urethral recurrence developed presented with a change in voiding habits, which in one case was the patient's only complaint [32]. One should consider a urethral recurrence in the differential diagnosis whenever a patient who has undergone lower urinary tract reconstruction with an orthotopic neobladder presents with a change in voiding habits.

Treatment of urethral transitional cell carcinoma after radical cystectomy

The ideal treatment for a urethral recurrence after radical cystectomy remains a total urethrectomy. Attempts to perform subtotal (meatus sparing) urethrectomies have been abandoned owing to documented reports of late recurrences at the urethral meatus [4,13,15,19,21,34]. As many as 27% of patients with a urethral recurrence after cystectomy who undergo a total urethrectomy will have involvement of the glanular urethra [21]. In a review of the data from a cohort of 1054 patients with more than 10-year median follow-up, two patients were identified who had undergone en bloc subtotal urethrectomy at the time of radical cystectomy with later recurrences at the urethral meatus 3 and 11 years after cystectomy (J. P. Stein, MD, personal communication, May 15, 2002). Both of these patients required surgical excision (one via distal penectomy and one via excision of the meatus). In patients with cutaneous diversion, standard treatment of urethral TCC should be a total urethrectomy including excision of the meatus.

For selected patients in whom urethral TCC develops after an orthotopic diversion, an attempt at endoscopic management with or without the instillation of intravesical therapy has been attempted. A recent study reported success using a regimen of intraurethral instillation of 5-fluorouracil in one of three patients [32]. In another study, a patient with CIS of the urethra after definitive radiation for TCC of the bladder was treated with intraurethral instillations of bacillus Calmette-Guérin, which ultimately failed [55]. Given the limited experience with this approach, it should be entertained in highly selected patients only after fully discussing the risks involved.

Survival after urethral transitional cell carcinoma following radical cystectomy

Bladder versus urethral stage and outcome

Urethral recurrence is a potentially lethal disease. Patients in whom urethral recurrence develops after radical cystectomy have relatively poor median overall and disease-specific survival [19,32,33]. A recent report analyzing the outcomes among 47 patients with urethral TCC after radical cystectomy found that the median survival was 28 months [32]. The most important predictor of overall survival in that series was the stage of the urethral TCC at the time of diagnosis. Patients with invasive TCC of the urethra had significantly worse overall survival than patients with superficial disease (pTa) or CIS alone. The bladder stage at the time of cystectomy did not influence survival. Contrary to these findings, another study by Lin et al [56] found that, among 24 men who had undergone urethrectomy after radical cystectomy, only the cystectomy pathologic stage (not urethral stage) predicted overall survival. The reason for this contrast is most likely explained by differences in the patient population between the two studies. In the study by Clark et al, patients who were pT0 at the time of urethrectomy were excluded, and 42% of the patients had invasive disease [32]. In the study by Lin et al, 37% of the patients were pT0, and only 12.5% had invasive disease [56].

Evidence in the literature regarding the relative influence of bladder pathology versus urethral pathology on overall and disease-specific survival is sparse and contradictory. Most studies make no direct comparison between the relative influence of urethral versus bladder pathology or use historical controls. Nevertheless, several studies have suggested that patients with invasive or "overt" urethral recurrences have a poor outcome [14, 17,22,57]. Another study that compared outcomes based on the extent of invasion was by performed by Hendry et al [22]. These researchers compared the outcome among 20 patients and found that the mean survivals in those with CIS of the urethra versus invasive carcinoma were 44.8 and 5.1 months, respectively. No attempt was made to determine the significance of the differences noted, and no survival analysis was performed. Some studies suggest that patients with superficial urethral TCC at the time of recurrence do relatively well [3,14], whereas other studies have found a relatively poor outcome in patients with superficial urethral disease at the time of recurrence [16,37,58]. None of these studies contrasted the outcome among patients with invasive versus superficial disease. A study by Schellhammer and Whitmore concluded that survival was largely dependent on the stage and grade of the bladder tumor, whereas the relative influence of the urethral tumor was harder to define [4]; however, the study failed to delineate the data to support that argument. The relative influence of bladder versus urethral pathology on survival among patients with urethral TCC after radical cystectomy is difficult to determine with certainty and awaits further study. Ultimately, this determination may require pooling the experience from a number of large volume centers in an effort to increase the number of available patients for analysis.

Method of diagnosis and outcome

Relatively few studies have attempted to determine whether the method of diagnosis influences outcome among patients with a urethral recurrence. Several series have documented poor survival among patients with symptomatic urethral disease recurrence [4,23,34,38]. In one of the largest series to date, Schellhammer and Whitmore analyzed 27 patients with a symptomatic urethral recurrence after radical cystectomy for TCC [4]. Only four of these patients remained alive with no evidence of disease; 18 of the 27 died of metastatic TCC. Baron et al reported that 9 of their 12 patients with symptomatic urethral recurrences died of metastatic disease [34]. Several studies have looked at patients who had asymptomatic urethral recurrences diagnosed by cytology alone [3,17,20,40]. Hickey et al reviewed the records of seven patients diagnosed with asymptomatic urethral recurrences by cytology. All of these patients were found to have CIS on final pathology, and all subsequently remained free of disease [3]. Bardot and Montie examined nine

patients diagnosed with a urethral recurrence by cytology and reported that only one patient subsequently "died from urethral recurrence" [40]. None of these studies performed any comparative analyses.

Two early studies reported on patients with symptomatic and asymptomatic urethral recurrences [17,20]. A study by Ahlering et al found that, of six patients with an asymptomatic recurrence diagnosed by cytology, two (33%) later died of the disease, whereas 5 of 10 (50%) patients with a symptomatic urethral recurrence ultimately died of metastatic TCC [17]. The statistical significance of these findings was not explored in this small series of patients. Conversely, a smaller study by Faysal reported on eight patients with a urethral recurrence after cystectomy, half diagnosed by cytology alone and half presenting with symptoms [20]. Only one patient diagnosed by cytology was thought to have "possibly died of urethral recurrence." In addition, a study by Stockle et al analyzed 23 patients, the "majority" of whom were diagnosed by cytology. All 23 died of metastatic TCC [13]. A recent report analyzing 37 patients with urethral TCC after radical cystectomy found that the method of diagnosis did not influence survival (symptomatic diagnosis in 24 versus cytology alone in 13) [32]. Similarly, a recent study of 24 patients with urethral TCC found no difference in survival in a comparison of those who were followed up with (n = 17) or without (n = 7) routine urethral wash cytology [56]. Although the latter two studies are among the largest in the literature, they are still hampered by small numbers. The evidence in the literature is contradictory and limited by small numbers and comparisons across studies and historical controls.

A note on orthotopic diversion

Despite the poor overall prognosis in patients with a urethral recurrence after radical cystectomy, the percentage of patients in whom a recurrence develops is small. The reported rate in the literature is approximately 8% [26,31]. If all of the risk factors proposed to date for urethral recurrence were to serve as contraindications to orthotopic diversion, approximately 70% of patients would be ineligible [26]. When en bloc prophylactic urethrectomies are performed, 57% to 100% of the time no urethral TCC is identified [4,9–11,13,14,16,20,59,60]. Furthermore, at least two studies have found no difference in outcome when comparing patients with or without prophylactic urethrectomy at the time of cystectomy [18,22]. Indeed, as discussed previously, there is at least one report suggesting that patients with an orthotopic diversion have a lower urethral recurrence rate than patients with an incontinent or continent cutaneous diversion [26]. This observation suggests there may be an unidentified protective influence of the native urethra when there is ongoing voiding from a neobladder. The disappointing survival among patients with urethral TCC after radical cystectomy does not mean that patients cannot undergo orthotopic diversion; rather, it suggests that the procedure can be performed safely in properly selected patients with a negative urethral margin on frozen section at the time of radical cystectomy. It is imperative that the surgeon and patient be committed to life-long follow-up of the native urethra, including annual cytologic examination, investigation of any symptoms (including any change in voiding habits), and aggressive management should a recurrence be diagnosed.

Summary

The incidence of urethral TCC after radical cystectomy is approximately 8% overall. The most important risk factor for urethral TCC after radical cystectomy and urinary diversion is prostatic involvement by TCC, particularly stromal invasion. The safety of using the urethra for orthotopic urinary diversion seems to be best when intraoperative frozen section analysis of the urethral margin is performed at the time of radical cystectomy. There is provocative but unconfirmed evidence that orthotopic urinary diversion may be protective against the development of urethral TCC. Although most urethral "recurrences" occur within 5 years, delayed recurrences have been documented, mandating life-long follow-up of the retained urethra. Follow-up should include urinary cytology, either voided or urethral wash cytology as appropriate, with evaluation by endoscopy of any urethral related symptoms or change in voiding symptoms. The management of urethral TCC after cystectomy remains a total urethrectomy including excision of the meatus; however, in carefully selected patients with superficial disease and an orthotopic urinary diversion, urethra sparing may be attempted after a careful discussion with the patient. Survival after urethral TCC has generally been disappointing. The relative value of urethral versus original cystectomy pathologic stage and

symptomatic versus nonsymptomatic recurrence in predicting survival remains controversial and awaits further studies that will most likely require the pooling of data from several large series.

References

[1] Jemal A, Tiwari RC, Murray T, et al. Cancer statistics, 2004. CA Cancer J Clin 2004;54(1):8–29.

[2] Messing EM, Catalona W. Urothelial tumors of the urinary tract. In: Walsh PC, Retik AB, Vaughan EDJ, editors. Campbell's urology, vol. 3. 7th edition. Philadelphia: WB Saunders; 1998. p. 2327–410.

[3] Hickey DP, Soloway MS, Murphy WM. Selective urethrectomy following cystoprostatectomy for bladder cancer. J Urol 1986;136(4):828–30.

[4] Schellhammer PF, Whitmore WF Jr. Transitional cell carcinoma of the urethra in men having cystectomy for bladder cancer. J Urol 1976;115(1):56–60.

[5] Skinner DG, Stein JP, Lieskovsky G, et al. 25-Year experience in the management of invasive bladder cancer by radical cystectomy. Eur Urol 1998; 33(Suppl 4):25–6.

[6] Kitamura T, Moriyama N, Shibamoto K, et al. Urethrectomy is harmful for preserving potency after radical cystectomy. Urol Int 1987;42(5):375–9.

[7] Tomic R, Sjodin JG. Sexual function in men after radical cystectomy with or without urethrectomy. Scand J Urol Nephrol 1992;26(2):127–9.

[8] Lilien OM, Camey M. 25-Year experience with replacement of the human bladder (Camey procedure). J Urol 1984;132:886.

[9] Freeman JA, Esrig D, Stein JP, et al. Management of the patient with bladder cancer: urethral recurrence. Urol Clin North Am 1994;21(4):645–51.

[10] Tobisu K, Tanaka Y, Mizutani T, et al. Transitional cell carcinoma of the urethra in men following cystectomy for bladder cancer: multivariate analysis for risk factors. J Urol 1991;146(6):1551–3; discussion, 1553–4.

[11] Levinson AK, Johnson DE, Wishnow KI. Indications for urethrectomy in an era of continent urinary diversion. J Urol 1990;144(1):73–5.

[12] Hardeman SW, Soloway MS. Urethral recurrence following radical cystectomy. J Urol 1990;144(3): 666–9.

[13] Stockle M, Gokcebay E, Riedmiller H, et al. Urethral tumor recurrences after radical cystoprostatectomy: the case for primary cystoprostatourethrectomy? J Urol 1990;143(1):41–2; discussion, 43.

[14] Nurmi M, Puntala P, Ekfors T. Urethral recurrence after cystoprostatectomy for bladder carcinoma. Scand J Urol Nephrol 1989;23(1):1–2.

[15] Shinka T, Uekado Y, Aoshi H, et al. Urethral remnant tumors following simultaneous partial urethrectomy and cystectomy for bladder carcinoma. J Urol 1989;142(4):983–7.

[16] Lopez-Almansa M, Molina R, Huben RP. Transitional cell carcinoma of the urethra in men after radical cystectomy for bladder cancer: is prophylactic urethrectomy indicated? Br J Urol 1988;61(6):507–9.

[17] Ahlering TA, Lieskovsky G, Skinner DG. Indications for urethrectomy in men undergoing single stage radical cystectomy for bladder cancer. J Urol 1984;131:657.

[18] Beahrs JR, Fleming TR, Zincke H. Risk of local urethral recurrence after radical cystectomy for bladder cancer. J Urol 1984;131(2):264–6.

[19] Zabbo A, Montie JE. Management of the urethra in men undergoing radical cystectomy for bladder cancer. J Urol 1984;131(2):267–8.

[20] Faysal MH. Urethrectomy in men with transitional cell carcinoma of bladder. Urology 1980;16(1):23–6.

[21] Schellhammer PF, Whitmore WF Jr. Urethral meatal carcinoma following cystourethrectomy for bladder cancer. J Urol 1976;115:61–4.

[22] Hendry WF, Gowing NFC, Wallace DM. Surgical treatment of urethral tumors associated with bladder cancer. Proc R Soc Med 1974;67:304–7.

[23] Cordonnier JJ, Spjut HJ. Urethral occurrence of bladder carcinoma following cystectomy. J Urol 1962;87:398–403.

[24] Gowing NFC. Urethral carcinoma associated with cancer of the bladder. Br J Urol 1960;32:428–38.

[25] Ashworth A. Papillomatosis of the urethra. Br J Urol 1956;28:3–11.

[26] Freeman JA, Tarter TA, Esrig D, et al. Urethral recurrence in patients with orthotopic ileal neobladders. J Urol 1996;156(5):1615–9.

[27] Lebret T, Herve JM, Barre P, et al. Urethral recurrence of transitional cell carcinoma of the bladder: predictive value of preoperative latero-montanal biopsies and urethral frozen sections during prostatocystectomy. Eur Urol 1998;33(2):170–4.

[28] Robert M, Burgel JS, Serre I, et al. Les recidives urethrales apres cysto-prostatectomie pour tumeur vesicale. Progres en Urologie 1996;6(4):558–63.

[29] Slaton JW, Swanson DA, Grossman HB, et al. A stage specific approach to tumor surveillance after radical cystectomy for transitional cell carcinoma of the bladder. J Urol 1999;162(3 Pt 1):710–4.

[30] Steven K, Poulsen AL. The orthotopic Kock ileal neobladder: functional results, urodynamic features, complications and survival in 166 men. J Urol 2000;164(2):288–95.

[31] Stenzl A, Bartsch G, Rogatsch H. The remnant urothelium after reconstructive bladder surgery. Eur Urol 2002;41(2):124–31.

[32] Clark PE, Stein JP, Groshen SG, et al. The management of urethral transitional cell carcinoma after radical cystectomy for invasive bladder cancer. J Urol 2004;172(4 Pt 1):1342–7.

[33] Poole-Wilson DS, Barnard RJ. Total cystectomy for bladder tumours. Br J Urol 1971;43:16–24.

[34] Baron JC, Gibod LB, Steg A. Management of the urethra in patients undergoing radical cystectomy for bladder carcinoma. Eur Urol 1989;16:283–5.

[35] Erckert M, Stenzl A, Falk M, et al. Incidence of urethral tumour involvement in 910 men with bladder cancer. World J Urol 1996;14:3–8.

[36] Tongaonkar HB, Dalal AV, Kulkarni JN, et al. Urethral recurrences following radical cystectomy for invasive transitional cell carcinoma of the bladder. Br J Urol 1993;72(6):910–4.

[37] Richie JP, Skinner DG. Carcinoma in situ of the urethra associated with bladder carcinoma: the role of urethrectomy. J Urol 1978;119:80–1.

[38] Clark PB. Urethral carcinoma after cystectomy: the case for routine urethrectomy. J Urol (Paris) 1984;90:173–5.

[39] Tobisu K, Kanai Y, Sakamoto M, et al. Involvement of the anterior urethra in male patients with transitional cell-carcinoma of the bladder undergoing radical cystectomy with simultaneous urethrectomy. Jpn J Clin Oncol 1997;27(6):406–9.

[40] Bardot SF, Montie JE. Urethral recurrence after cystoprostatectomy. J Urol 1991;145(suppl):338A.

[41] Bell CR, Gujral S, Collins CM, et al. The fate of the urethra after definitive treatment of invasive transitional cell carcinoma of the urinary bladder. BJU Int 1999;83(6):607–12.

[42] Van Poppel H, Sorgeloose T. Radical cystectomy with or without urethrectomy? Crit Rev Oncol Hematol 2003;47(2):141–5.

[43] Hautmann RE, Paiss T, de Petriconi R. The ileal neobladder in women: 9 years of experience with 18 patients. J Urol 1996;155(1):76–81.

[44] Cancrini A, De Carli P, Fattahi H, et al. Orthotopic ileal neobladder in female patients after radical cystectomy: 2-year experience. J Urol 1995;153(3 Pt 2):956–8.

[45] Jarolim L, Babjuk M, Hanus T, et al. Female urethra-sparing cystectomy and orthotopic bladder replacement. Eur Urol 1997;31(2):173–7.

[46] Tobisu K, Coloby PJ, Fujimoto H, et al. An ileal neobladder for a female patient after a radical cystectomy to ensure voiding from the urethra: a case report. Jpn J Clin Oncol 1992;22(5):359–64.

[47] Stein JP, Stenzl A, Esrig D, et al. Lower urinary tract reconstruction following cystectomy in women using the Kock ileal reservoir with bilateral ureteroileal urethrostomy: initial clinical experience. J Urol 1994;152(5 Pt 1):1404–8.

[48] Stenzl A, Colleselli K, Poisel S, et al. Anterior exenteration with subsequent ureteroileal urethrostomy in females: anatomy, risk of urethral recurrence, surgical technique, and results. Eur Urol 1998;33(Suppl 4):18–20.

[49] Stenzl A, Draxl H, Posch B, et al. The risk of urethral tumors in female bladder cancer: can the urethra be

used for orthotopic reconstruction of the lower urinary tract? J Urol 1995;153(3 Pt 2):950–5.

[50] Coloby PJ, Kakizoe T, Tobisu K, et al. Urethral involvement in female bladder cancer patients: mapping of 47 consecutive cysto-urethrectomy specimens. J Urol 1994;152(5 Pt 1):1438–42.

[51] Stein JP, Esrig D, Freeman JA, et al. Prospective pathologic analysis of female cystectomy specimens: risk factors for orthotopic diversion in women. Urology 1998;51(6):951–5.

[52] Stenzl A, Colleselli K, Poisel S, et al. The use of neobladders in women undergoing cystectomy for transitional-cell cancer. World J Urol 1996;14(1):15–21.

[53] Jones J, Melchior SW, Gillitzer R, et al. Urethral recurrence of transitional cell carcinoma in a female patient after cystectomy and orthotopic ileal neobladder. J Urol 2000;164(5):1646.

[54] Wolinska WH, Melamed MR, Schellhammer PF, et al. Urethral cytology following cystectomy for bladder carcinoma. Am J Surg Pathol 1977;1:225.

[55] Witjes JA, Debruyne FM, van der Meijden AP. Treatment of carcinoma in situ of the urethra with intraurethral instillations of bacillus Calmette-Guerin: case report and review of literature. Eur Urol 1991;20(2):170–2.

[56] Lin DW, Herr HW, Dalbagni G. Value of urethral wash cytology in the retained male urethra after radical cystoprostatectomy. J Urol 2003;169(3):961–3.

[57] Raz S, McLorie G, Johnson S, et al. Management of the urethra in patients undergoing radical cystectomy for bladder carcinoma. J Urol 1978;120:298–300.

[58] Cheville JC, Dundore PA, Bostwick DG, et al. Transitional cell carcinoma of the prostate: clinicopathologic study of 50 cases. Cancer 1998;82(4):703–7.

[59] Coutts AG, Grigor KM, Fowler JW. Urethral dysplasia and bladder cancer in cystectomy specimens. Br J Urol 1985;57:535–41.

[60] Stams UK, Gursel EO, Veenema RJ. Prophylactic urethrectomy in male patients with bladder cancer. J Urol 1974;111:177–9.

ELSEVIER
SAUNDERS

Urol Clin N Am 32 (2005) 207–216

UROLOGIC
CLINICS
of North America

Quality of Life Issues in Bladder Cancer Patients Following Cystectomy and Urinary Diversion

Michael P. Porter, MD, MSE[a], John T. Wei, MD, MSE[b],
David F. Penson, MD, MPH[c],*

[a]Department of Urology, University of Washington, H220 Health Sciences Center,
Box 357183, Seattle, WA 98195-7183, USA
[b]Department of Urology, University of Michigan, 1500 E. Medical Center Drive,
Womens Trailer Room 1013, Ann Arbor, MI 48109-0759, USA
[c]Departments of Urology and Preventative Medicine, Keck School of Medicine,
University of Southern California, 1441 Eastlake Avenue, Suite 7416,
Los Angeles, CA 90089, USA

Radical cystectomy with urinary diversion is currently the standard therapy for invasive bladder cancer. In the past, noncontinent conduit diversion was the primary form of urinary tract reconstruction, but with the introduction of continent orthotopic diversions, options for reconstruction have increased. With experience, it has been shown that patients undergoing continent forms of urinary diversion have similar perioperative complication rates, cancer control, and survival to patients undergoing conduit diversions [1–3]. It has been estimated that 80% of men and 65% of women with invasive bladder cancer are candidates for an orthotopic neobladder [4].

When different treatments for the same disease offer similar cancer control and disease-specific and overall survival, quality of life becomes a crucial endpoint when critically comparing therapies. Additionally, it has been recognized that the length of survival, although important,

needs to be interpreted in the context of quality of life. Health-related quality of life (HRQOL) is a variable from the field of health services research that has been defined as the value assigned by individuals, groups, or society to the duration of survival modified by impairments, functional states, perceptions, and social opportunities influenced by disease, injury, or treatment [5]. More concisely, it is a measure of the patient's evaluation of the impact of a health condition and its treatments on relevant aspects of life. Knowledge of HRQOL allows physicians and patients to better understand expected outcomes of illness and therapy, providing the information needed to make more informed decisions regarding the most appropriate treatment for an individual patient.

For the reasons outlined previously, invasive bladder cancer is a disease in which knowledge of HRQOL is important; however, understanding of HRQOL outcomes in patients who undergo cystectomy and urinary diversion for bladder cancer is still in its earliest stages. This review outlines HRQOL issues in patients undergoing cystectomy and urinary diversion for bladder cancer and summarizes the current state of the evidence. This review not only focuses on what is currently known based on the published literature but also briefly outlines methods of measuring HRQOL, challenges in measuring HRQOL in bladder cancer patients, and future directions for research.

Dr. Porter is a Robert Wood Johnson Clinical Scholar whose position is supported financially by the Veteran's Administration. The opinions in this article represent those of the authors and not necessarily those of the Robert Wood Johnson Foundation or the Veteran's Administration.

* Corresponding author.
 E-mail address: penson@usc.edu (D.F. Penson).

Measuring health-related quality of life

Many questionnaires are available to measure generic HRQOL. Whether administered by an interviewer or self-reported by the patient, all HRQOL questionnaires (or instruments) attempt to measure relevant aspects of the impact of illness and treatment from the patient's perspective. These relevant aspects are measured as domains. Commonly measured domains include symptoms, psychologic impact, physical impact, and social impact of the illness. HRQOL instruments can be generic (sometimes referred to as general) or disease specific. Generic instruments are applicable to all patients, regardless of their illness, whereas disease-specific instruments focus on areas of quality of life that are specifically important to individuals with that particular disease state. For example, energy, stamina, and physical function apply to all individuals and are considered generic HRQOL, whereas urinary leakage, sexual function, and body image are most likely of particular interest to patients receiving treatment for invasive bladder cancer and are disease specific. Generic and disease-specific HRQOL instruments consist of multiple questions that are interrelated to form domains.

During development, HRQOL instruments should undergo a process of psychometric and clinical testing to establish their clinical usefulness. The development process is complex and beyond the scope of this article, but the ideal instrument should be valid (measures what it reports to measure), reliable (able to give the same result on several occasions given stable disease), and responsive (able to detect true but clinically meaningful changes). The generic term that is often used to describe an instrument that has undergone some form of developmental testing is "validated," but this term can be deceiving. Ideally, if an instrument is described as validated, it has undergone enough developmental testing that its validity, reliability, and responsiveness can be described quantitatively and are appropriate for the application of interest. Unfortunately, the term *validated* is often used loosely by investigators unfamiliar with health services research and does not always indicate that an instrument has undergone rigorous developmental testing commensurate to the application of interest.

Generic HRQOL instruments are applied across different diseases, conditions, populations, and concepts [6]. Examples of generic instruments are the SF-36 [7], the Quality of Well-Being scale [8], and the Sickness Impact Profile (SIP) [9]. Each of these instruments has undergone extensive developmental testing and is considered a valid and reliable instrument to measure HRQOL. Because generic instruments measure HRQOL independent of a specific disease or treatment, they are broadly applicable and lend themselves to easy comparison of HRQOL across different diseases and treatments; however, this lack of specificity may limit their responsiveness to change. For example, the SF-36 does not include items on sexual function. If it were used to measure HRQOL in a disease in which erectile dysfunction was a major sequelae, it may not be sufficiently sensitive to capture relevant changes in HRQOL.

Disease-specific instruments attempt to measure HRQOL as it pertains to a specific disease or its therapy. They include items that may be specific to the illness of interest, such as urinary incontinence and sexual function for genitourinary diseases. Disease-specific instruments are generally more responsive to expected changes associated with the disease of interest, but their specificity may make them less likely to detect unanticipated effects. For example, if a treatment has an unanticipated gastrointestinal side effect, and the HRQOL instrument being used does not include items for that domain, it may not accurately assess HRQOL changes associated with the therapy. Their specificity for a particular disease also makes it difficult to use their results to compare HRQOL across different diseases.

Multiple instruments are available to assess cancer-specific HRQOL. Two examples are the European Organization for Research and Treatment of Cancer-QOL (EORTC-QLQ-C30) [10] and the Functional Assessment of Cancer Therapy general form (FACT-G) [11]. Both of these instruments include items that are germane to cancer therapy, such as gastrointestinal side effects, energy level, and mood. Both of these instruments have also undergone extensive testing and are considered valid and reliable measures of HRQOL in cancer patients. Although they are more specific than generic instruments, cancer-specific instruments may not be specific enough to respond to HRQOL changes that occur in bladder cancer patients after cystectomy and urinary diversion.

Currently, few disease-specific instruments are available to measure HRQOL in bladder cancer patients who require cystectomy and urinary diversion. The FACT-BL is an adaptation of the

FACT-G that includes 12 additional items specific to bladder cancer, including items on incontinence, diarrhea, body image, sexual function, and stoma care. The FACT-BL has been reported as validated [12]; however, the authors could not find published validation studies in a PubMed search. The EORTC-QLQ-BLM30 is an adaptation of the EORTC-QLQ-C30 and contains 30 additional items specific to bladder cancer. The EORTC-QLQ-BLM30 is in phase 3 of 4 of the EORTC development protocol (N. Aaronson, personal communication, 2004). It has completed pretesting but still needs to complete large-scale field testing before it can be considered validated. Other efforts are underway to validate bladder cancer–specific instruments. Specifically, in 2003, Cookson et al [13] reported the results of an initial validation study of a bladder cancer–specific instrument, the Vanderbilt cystectomy index (FACT-VCI). The instrument was designed to measure HRQOL in patients who underwent radical cystectomy and urinary diversion for bladder cancer. The developers combined the FACT-G with 17 additional bladder cancer–specific items, some of which are also included in the FACT-BL. The initial validation study on 50 patients was promising, but this instrument is also in its early stages of development.

Challenges when measuring health-related quality of life in bladder cancer patients with urinary diversion

Measuring HRQOL in patients with bladder cancer and urinary diversion poses unique challenges. The first and most obvious is the issue of sexual dysfunction. Because bladder cancer affects men and women, and because radical cystectomy affects sexual function for men and women in potentially different ways, designing a single instrument that captures these effects in both genders is difficult. Numerous complicated domains must be considered when assessing sexuality in bladder cancer patients. For example, one could consider penile erections in men, orgasmic function, libido, and body image, among others. The issue of assessing sexual domains following cystectomy is further complicated by the differential sexual impact that surgery has on women and men. Problems with vaginal lubrication, vaginal shortening, and changes in perineal and vaginal sensation are all problems unique to women. Capturing the impact of these issues in a single instrument designed to be administered to men and women is difficult, and the results are likely to be unique to each sex. It is likely that the impact of cystectomy on sexual domains will be very different between the sexes and only comparable among patients of the same sex unless comparable items are developed and validated.

As difficult as it is to measure HRQOL issues in the sexual domain among cystectomy patients, it is likely to be even more challenging to measure changes in the urinary domain. Common items designed to capture changes in the urinary domain include questions about frequency, urgency, and incontinence. Nevertheless, these standard items are unlikely to capture the nuances that may be unique to each diversion. Problems with stoma appliances, the use of catheters, incontinence, day and nighttime leakage, and urinary tract infection are likely to be different depending on the type of diversion. This task may be complicated further by a differential impact of such problems between the sexes. For example, urethral catheterization is a different experience for men than it is for women, and this may translate into an HRQOL difference. The impact on body image that occurs with different types of stomas and external appliances may also be different for men than for women. Further complicating the issue, different diversions may lead to different symptoms unrelated to the urinary domain, such as diarrhea and metabolic abnormalities. Capturing and characterizing the impact of all these factors on HRQOL in a manner that is responsive to change and generalizable among different types of diversion is a challenging task that will not be easy for researchers to overcome.

The final set of challenges is not unique to bladder cancer. Problems associated with study design and generalizability plague all clinical research but may be particularly difficult to overcome in assessing HRQOL in bladder cancer patients requiring cystectomy. A randomized multicenter study that enrolled bladder cancer patients of all ages and that encompassed the entire range of health statuses would be the optimal choice of study design to compare HRQOL following various urinary diversions. Unfortunately, HRQOL studies tend to occur at academic centers where patient populations are often not representative of bladder cancer patients at large. Furthermore, although bladder cancer is relatively common, it would be difficult to accrue adequate numbers of subjects to a randomized study given patient and provider biases. Bladder cancer also tends to be a disease of the elderly; therefore, it is reasonable to speculate that this population of patients is least likely to experience HRQOL differences based on different types of diversion, because comorbidities and physical limitations may overwhelm any differences that exist. Results from studies in this age group may not be generalizable to younger bladder cancer patients who may have more to gain in HRQOL with a continent or orthotopic diversion. Although challenging, this final set of problems should be the easiest to overcome with proper planning and study design.

Health-related quality of life in bladder cancer patients after cystectomy

Multiple studies have been published that examine HRQOL in patients after cystectomy and urinary diversion for bladder cancer. Unfortunately, many of these studies have employed differing methods, used different instruments, and compared different diversions. Not surprisingly, the results from these studies are conflicting and, on balance, are difficult to interpret. In effort to clarify the current state of the evidence, two of the authors (MPP, DFP) recently published a systematic review of the literature to identify research articles addressing quality of life after cystectomy and urinary diversion for bladder cancer [14].

Briefly, a MEDLINE search was performed inclusive of the dates 1966 to January 2004 to identify studies comparing HRQOL outcomes between different types of urinary diversion for bladder cancer. The following search terms were used: neobladder AND quality of life; continent reservoir AND quality of life; ileal conduit AND quality of life; urinary diversion AND quality of life; urinary conduit AND quality of life; and urinary diversion AND health-related quality of life. The individual results of each of the searches were then pooled, resulting in 378 unique articles. Articles were excluded that did not exclusively address bladder cancer patients, that included patients who received radiotherapy, or that did not compare at least two of the following types of urinary diversion: ileal conduit, orthotopic neobladder, or continent cutaneous urinary reservoir. Fifteen publications met all of these criteria [15–29] and are summarized in Table 1.

Two major findings arose from this systematic review. First, only one study was performed prospectively and included baseline data before the cystectomy as well as data after the surgery [22]. This study was performed in Germany and collected preoperative baseline HRQOL data on 20 patients undergoing continent cutaneous reservoirs and 24 patients undergoing ileal conduits. Follow-up HRQOL was measured at 2 to 4 weeks and 12 months postoperatively. Using two generic and one unvalidated disease-specific HRQOL instruments, the researchers found that HRQOL returned to baseline at 1 year, regardless of diversion. They also found that conduit patients required appliance emptying more often then did patients with reservoirs, and that reservoir patients were more likely to sustain diarrhea. The remaining studies were retrospective and cross-sectional, with the instrument administered at a single point in time months to years after surgery.

Second, many of the studies (10/15) used unvalidated instruments to measure bladder cancer–specific HRQOL. Most of the unvalidated instruments were attempts at capturing relevant disease-specific domains for cystectomy patients and were mostly ad hoc questionnaires developed by the investigators and administered without any prior validation attempts. When validated instruments were used, they tended to be generic or cancer specific and, for the reasons previously described, may not have been responsive to changes unique to patients with cystectomy and urinary diversion.

Despite these methodologic problems, some common themes arose from the 15 studies. Three studies indicated that patients with a conduit diversion had more difficulties with urine leakage than did patients with a form of continent diversion [15,17,27]. The most recent of these studies was reported by Bjerre et al in 1995 [15]. These investigators compared 29 patients with an ileal conduit with 38 patients with a urethral Kock reservoir, all of who were recruited from three centers in Denmark. Using an unvalidated instrument, they found that a statistically significant higher proportion of ileal conduit patients (58% versus 21%) reported urinary leakage as their main concern.

Three studies indicated that patients with a continent form of diversion were more likely to travel than were patients with a conduit [24,25,29]. The most recent of these studies was reported by Hobisch et al [24]. These researchers used the EORTC-QLC-C30 and an unvalidated bladder cancer–specific instrument to compare 69 patients with an orthotopic neobladder with

33 patients with an ileal conduit. One of the main findings was that leisure activities and travel were reduced by a statistically significant amount (8.7% versus 36.4% and 21.7% versus 51.5%, respectively) in the ileal conduit patients. Although these studies suggest a possible effect of diversion type on patient activities, such differences may also be explained by selection bias (eg, if more active patients are more likely to choose a continent diversion over an ileal conduit).

Two studies indicated that patients with continent diversions were more likely to report a better quality of life in the social/emotional domains [18,23]. The larger of these studies, reported by Hart et al [23], compared 25 patients with an ileal conduit, 93 patients with a cutaneous Kock pouch, and 103 patients with a urethral Kock pouch. Although most of the HRQOL domains were similar, ileal conduit patients were more likely to report a worse HRQOL in the social domains than were cutaneous or orthotopic diversion patients. Eleven of the fifteen studies reported that HRQOL outcomes were equivalent in all or most of the domains measured. These observations may provide some insight into HRQOL issues facing bladder cancer patients with urinary diversion and provide a framework of issues to consider when designing future studies or HRQOL instruments.

Two other recent reviews examined the literature on HRQOL after cystectomy in bladder cancer patients. In 2003, Botteman et al [12] reported the results of a large structured review examining HRQOL in bladder cancer patients. The review was not limited to bladder cancer patients requiring cystectomy. Nevertheless, the researchers did focus some of their efforts on this topic, and they reached conclusions similar to those just outlined. They concluded that the literature on this topic was extensive but was limited by suboptimal methods, including design problems, small sample sizes, retrospective data, and insensitive and unvalidated instruments. They also concluded that, although HRQOL decreases after urinary diversion, it does not decrease dramatically, and the decrease occurs principally in the sexual and urinary domains. The very limited evidence available to date using poorly validated instruments did not support one form of urinary diversion over another. Each diversion was associated with its own set of symptoms and impact on HRQOL, such as a decrease in body image in conduit diversion, symptoms related to catheter use in continent reservoirs, and

symptoms related to nocturnal incontinence in neobladder patients. Based on their review, Botteman and colleagues concluded that no one type of diversion was superior in terms of HRQOL, and that the best course of action may be to match individual patients with the most appropriate diversion based on patient preference and known morbidities.

More recently, Parkinson and Konety [30] reviewed the literature pertaining to HRQOL assessment in bladder cancer patients. When they examined the published literature pertaining to HRQOL after cystectomy and urinary diversion, their conclusions were similar to that of the authors. They concluded that most of the studies had methodologic problems, including a lack of prospective data collection. Most of the studies showed equivalent HRQOL among different types of urinary diversion, including conduit diversion. Each diversion was associated with a specific set of symptoms that had the potential to affect HRQOL, but the currently published studies had not demonstrated that that these symptoms were severe enough to change HRQOL.

Based on the three reviews of the existing literature described herein, it seems reasonable to conclude that HRQOL has not been shown unequivocally to vary between the different types of urinary diversion in bladder cancer patients. As might be expected, the domains most affected by cystectomy and urinary diversion are urinary and sexual. Each type of diversion is associated with specific symptoms that may impact HRQOL; however, given the lack of well-validated instruments to capture these concerns, it is entirely possible that significant differences exist but have not yet been demonstrated. Based on the current knowledge of HRQOL, patients should be counseled on an individual basis regarding the expected symptoms and morbidity of each diversion, and a diversion should be chosen based on patient preference and not on the promise of a better HRQOL.

Future directions

Despite the commonly held belief by urologic surgeons that there are quality of life differences between various diversions after radical cystectomy for bladder cancer, the published literature does not conclusively document that one form of diversion is superior to another in terms of HRQOL. The lack of unambiguous evidence supporting an HRQOL advantage of continent forms of diversion is most

Table 1
Studies comparing HRQOL outcomes in bladder cancer patients undergoing cystectomy and urinary diversion

Study	Comparison (n)	Instrument — General or disease specific	Validated	Study design	Source population	Major findings
Bjerre et al (1995)	NB (38)	Specific	No	Retrospective	Denmark	Incontinence more bothersome in IC patients, other parameters equivalent
Boyd et al (1987)	IC (29) CR (85)	Specific	No	Cross-sectional Retrospective	United States	CR patients more likely to be sexually active, other parameters equivalent
	IC (87)	Specific (mental health) General (mental health)	Yes Yes	Cross-sectional		
Conde et al (2001)	NB (27)	Specific	No	Retrospective	Spain	IC patients had more problems with urine leakage and depression
	IC (6)			Cross-sectional		
Dutta et al (2002)	NB (49)	General	Yes	Retrospective	United States	NB better on several domains, but only marginal difference after adjusting for age, stage, and sex
Fujisawa et al (2000)	IC (23) NB (36) IC (20)	General (cancer) General	Yes Yes	Cross-sectional Retrospective Cross-sectional	Japan	No differences found
Gerharz et al (1997)	CR (64) IC (326)	Specific	No	Retrospective Cross-sectional	Germany	CR better in some domains and on stoma-related items, overall QOL equivalent
Hara et al (2002)	NB (48) IC (37)	General Specific	Yes No	Retrospective Cross-sectional	Japan	Equivalent in all domains of SF-36
Hardt et al (2000)	CR (20)	General	Yes	Prospective	Germany	Sexual function equivalent, all SF-36 domains returned to baseline by 1 year except physical function
	IC (24)	General Specific	Yes No	Longitudinal		

Study	Diversion (N)	Instrument		Design	Country	Findings
Hart et al (1999)	NB (103)	General (mental health)	Yes	Retrospective	United States	IC patients had worse social function
	CR (93)	General (sexual function)	No	Cross-sectional		
	IC (25)	General (body image)	No			
		General	No			
Hobisch et al (2001)	NB (69)	General (cancer)	Yes	Retrospective	Austria	NB better in all domains. NB with more travel and leisure and more likely to recommend to friend
Kitamura et al (1999)	IC (33)	Specific	No	Cross-sectional	Japan	IC patients more likely to have trouble with public restrooms and travel
	NB (21)	General (cancer)	Yes	Retrospective		
	CR (22)	Specific	No	Cross-sectional		
	IC (36)					
Mansson et al (1988)	CR (20)	Specific	No	Retrospective	Sweden	IC patients had more problems with leakage and odor, other parameters equivalent
	IC (40)			Cross-sectional		
Mansson et al (2002)	NB (29)	Specific (bladder cancer)	Yes	Retrospective	Sweden	NB had more difficulties with incontinence, FACT-G and HADS measures equivalent
McGuire et al (2000)	CR (35)	Specific (mental health)	Yes	Cross-sectional	United States	All groups equivalent when compared to population norms
	NB (38)	General	Yes	Retrospective		
	CR (16)			Cross-sectional		
	IC (38)					
Okada et al (1997)	CR (74)	Specific	No	Retrospective	Japan	CR bathed more, traveled more, and had less local stoma problems
	IC (63)			Cross-sectional		

Abbreviations: IC, ileal conduit; CR, continent reservoir; NB, neobladder.

likely the result of limitations in the existing literature and disease-specific HRQOL outcome measures, rather than true equivalence in HRQOL following various forms of continent urinary diversion. With some modifications in approach, it may be possible to answer these important questions more conclusively.

Study design

Nearly all of the published studies comparing quality of life outcomes in bladder cancer patients after urinary diversion are retrospective. In these studies, researchers identified patients long after surgery and administered an HRQOL instrument at a single point in time. This approach has several limitations. First, and perhaps most importantly, there is the problem of selection bias. Patients are often selected for a specific type of diversion based on the presence of comorbid disease and other clinical factors. In as much as these factors are also related to HRQOL, the results of a retrospective analysis that do not take this into account will be biased. Similarly, patient factors that influence the type of urinary diversion may also impact baseline preoperative HRQOL. If HRQOL is only measured at a point in time postoperatively, it is not possible to determine the amount that HRQOL changed owing to urinary diversion. This difference is arguably the main outcome of interest, and without baseline preoperative measurement of HRQOL, it cannot be determined.

Another problem with a retrospective approach is the variable time after surgery at which HRQOL is assessed. A patient 2 years removed from a cystectomy may have a different HRQOL than at 6 months, and this difference may be due solely to the adjustment to health status that occurs with time. In all but one of the studies listed in Table 1, patients with an ileal conduit were farther out from surgery than those with continent forms of diversion, raising the possibility of bias introduced by time.

A retrospective approach does not allow for longitudinal measurements of HRQOL. This drawback is related to the last point, because HRQOL is expected to change over the course of a disease. In fact, the only study listed in Table 1 that was performed prospectively found that HRQOL returned to baseline at 1 year postoperatively [22]. Repeated measurements over time would allow better characterization of HRQOL changes, and would allow potentially important comparisons in quality of life between

different types of urinary diversion that may occur at a time remote form surgery, such as near the end of life. Future observational studies should strive to overcome these limitations.

Health-related quality of life instruments

Another common limitation in studies performed to date is the use of unvalidated and often ad hoc instruments to measure HRQOL. As previously described, without proper validation, it is difficult to know whether the instruments are, in fact, measuring HRQOL, and how accurate the measurements are. Future studies should concentrate on using instruments with previous validation. Nevertheless, the main drawback to this approach is the lack of validated bladder cancer–specific instruments. Most of the published studies that relied on nonvalidated instruments did so in an attempt to capture bladder cancer–specific issues, such as stoma care, urinary leakage, and catheter use. The FACT-BL and the EORTC-QLQ-BLM30 bladder cancer–specific instruments have some degree of validation, and future instrument development should build on these efforts. It is hoped that experience will demonstrate that these and other emerging instruments are valid and reliable in HRQOL measurement for cystectomy patients. By combining these bladder cancer–specific instruments with generic instruments, it should be possible to capture HRQOL more accurately in this patient population.

Generalizability

Most of the current literature on HRQOL after urinary diversion in bladder cancer patients is a product of case series analysis from academic medical centers. Although this is not surprising, it poses potential problems in the generalizability of the results of these studies. First, patients referred to such centers may not be representative of the average bladder cancer patient. For example, disease severity and comorbidities may be different than in bladder cancer patients undergoing cystectomy in the community, and these factors may affect HRQOL outcomes. Second, differences in surgical technique, perioperative supportive care, and longer-term postoperative support may vary from center to center. Results from a series of 200 patients undergoing cystectomy by a single surgeon at a single center may and probably will vary from the results achieved by another surgeon at another center. Single institution case series need to be interpreted with caution, because

HRQOL outcomes may be dependent on factors that differ from institution to institution. Future studies should strive to be multicentered in nature.

Summary

HRQOL outcomes in bladder cancer patients undergoing cystectomy and urinary diversion are an important component in the critical assessment of bladder cancer treatment. To date, understanding of HRQOL in these patients remains poor. Although it is known that there are common factors that most likely affect HRQOL for all patients, it is unclear whether factors unique to a specific type of diversion impact HRQOL in a way that makes one type of diversion superior to another. Factors such as stoma maintenance, catheter use, urinary incontinence, body image, and sexual side effects are potentially different for each major type of diversion and most likely impact HRQOL, but a consistent advantage of one type of diversion over another has yet to be demonstrated. With slight changes in the approach to studying HRQOL outcomes, this question could be answered. Prospective study designs, appropriate adjustment for confounding factors, diverse patient populations, and the use of validated and disease-specific instruments would greatly enhance understanding of HRQOL in patients undergoing cystectomy for bladder cancer. By understating these issues more completely, patients could be counseled not only about their predicted surgical risks and survival but also about the impact their disease will have on their longer-term quality of survival. Patients will then be able to make a more fully informed decision on the most appropriate form of therapy for this serious life-altering disease.

References

[1] Clark PE. Urinary diversion after radical cystectomy. Curr Treat Options Oncol 2002;3(5):389–402.

[2] Krupski T, Theodorescu D. Orthotopic neobladder following cystectomy: indications, management, and outcomes. J Wound Ostomy Continence Nurs 2001;28(1):37–46.

[3] Madersbacher S, Studer UE. Contemporary cystectomy and urinary diversion. World J Urol 2002; 20(3):151–7.

[4] Hautmann RE. Which patients with transitional cell carcinoma of the bladder or prostatic urethra are candidates for an orthotopic neobladder? Curr Urol Rep 2000;1(3):173–9.

[5] Patrick DL, Erickson P. Health status and health policy: quality of life in health care evaluation and resource allocation. New York: Oxford University Press; 1993.

[6] Patrick DL, Chiang YP. Measurement of health outcomes in treatment effectiveness evaluations: conceptual and methodological challenges. Med Care 2000;38(9 Suppl): II14–25.

[7] Ware JE Jr, Sherbourne CD. The MOS 36-item short-form health survey (SF-36). I. Conceptual framework and item selection. Med Care 1992;30(6): 473–83.

[8] Kaplan RM, Anderson JP, Wu AW, et al. The Quality of Well-being Scale. Applications in AIDS, cystic, fibrosis, and arthritis. Med Care 1989; 27(3 Suppl):S27–43.

[9] Bergner M, Bobbitt RA, Carter WB, et al. The Sickness Impact Profile: development and final revision of a health status measure. Med Care 1981;19(8): 787–805.

[10] Aaronson NK, Ahmedzai S, Bergman B, et al. The European Organization for Research and Treatment of Cancer QLQ-C30: a quality-of-life instrument for use in international clinical trials in oncology. J Natl Cancer Inst 1993;85(5):365–76.

[11] Cella DF, Tulsky DS, Gray G, et al. The Functional Assessment of Cancer Therapy scale: development and validation of the general measure. J Clin Oncol 1993;11(3):570–9.

[12] Botteman MF, Pashos CL, Hauser RS, et al. Quality of life aspects of bladder cancer: a review of the literature. Qual Life Res 2003;12(6):675–88.

[13] Cookson MS, Dutta SC, Chang SS, et al. Health related quality of life in patients treated with radical cystectomy and urinary diversion for urothelial carcinoma of the bladder: development and validation of a new disease specific questionnaire. J Urol 2003;170(5):1926–30.

[14] Porter M, Penson DF. Health related quality of life after radical cystectomy and urinary diversion for bladder cancer: a systematic review and critical analysis of the literature. J Urol, in press.

[15] Bjerre BD, Johansen C, Steven K. Health-related quality of life after cystectomy: bladder substitution compared with ileal conduit diversion. A questionnaire survey. Br J Urol 1995;75(2):200–5.

[16] Boyd SD, Feinberg SM, Skinner DG, et al. Quality of life survey of urinary diversion patients: comparison of ileal conduits versus continent Kock ileal reservoirs. J Urol 1987;138(6):1386–9.

[17] Conde Redondo C, Estebanez Zarranz J, Rodriguez Tovez A, et al. [Quality of life in patients treated with orthotopic bladder substitution versus cutaneous ileostomy.] Actas Urol Esp 2001;25(6): 435–44.

[18] Dutta SC, Chang SC, Coffey CS, et al. Health related quality of life assessment after radical cystectomy: comparison of ileal conduit with continent orthotopic neobladder. J Urol 2002;168(1):164–7.

[19] Fujisawa M, Isotani S, Gotoh A, et al. Health-related quality of life with orthotopic neobladder

versus ileal conduit according to the SF-36 survey. Urology 2000;55(6):862–5.

[20] Gerharz EW, Weingartner K, Dopatka T, et al. Quality of life after cystectomy and urinary diversion: results of a retrospective interdisciplinary study. J Urol 1997;158(3 Pt 1):778–85.

[21] Hara I, Miyake H, Hara S, et al. Health-related quality of life after radical cystectomy for bladder cancer: a comparison of ileal conduit and orthotopic bladder replacement. BJU Int 2002;89(1):10–3.

[22] Hardt J, Filipas D, Hohenfellner R, et al. Quality of life in patients with bladder carcinoma after cystectomy: first results of a prospective study. Qual Life Res 2000;9(1):1–12.

[23] Hart S, Skinner EC, Meyerowitz BE, et al. Quality of life after radical cystectomy for bladder cancer in patients with an ileal conduit, cutaneous or urethral Kock pouch. J Urol 1999;162(1):77–81.

[24] Hobisch A, Tosun K, Kinzl J, et al. Life after cystectomy and orthotopic neobladder versus ileal conduit urinary diversion. Semin Urol Oncol 2001;19(1):18–23.

[25] Kitamura H, Miyao N, Yanase M, et al. Quality of life in patients having an ileal conduit, continent reservoir or orthotopic neobladder after cystectomy for bladder carcinoma. Int J Urol 1999;6(8):393–9.

[26] Mansson A, Davidsson T, Hunt S, et al. The quality of life in men after radical cystectomy with a continent cutaneous diversion or orthotopic bladder substitution: is there a difference? BJU Int 2002;90(4):386–90.

[27] Mansson A, Johnson G, Mansson W. Quality of life after cystectomy: comparison between patients with conduit and those with continent caecal reservoir urinary diversion. Br J Urol 1988;62(3):240–5.

[28] McGuire MS, Grimaldi G, Grotas J, et al. The type of urinary diversion after radical cystectomy significantly impacts on the patient's quality of life. Ann Surg Oncol 2000;7(1):4–8.

[29] Okada Y, Oishi K, Shichiri Y, et al. Quality of life survey of urinary diversion patients: comparison of continent urinary diversion versus ileal conduit. Int J Urol 1997;4(1):26–31.

[30] Parkinson JP, Konety BR. Health related quality of life assessments for patients with bladder cancer. J Urol 2004;172(6 Pt 1):2130–6.

ELSEVIER
SAUNDERS

Urol Clin N Am 32 (2005) 217–230

UROLOGIC
CLINICS
of North America

The Current and Future Application of Adjuvant Systemic Chemotherapy in Patients with Bladder Cancer Following Cystectomy

Ana M. Aparicio, MD, Anthony B. Elkhouiery, MD,
David I. Quinn, MD, PhD*

*Division of Medical Oncology and Kenneth J. Norris Comprehensive Cancer Center,
University of Southern California Keck School of Medicine, 1441 Eastlake Avenue, Los Angeles, CA 90089, USA*

Urothelial transitional cell cancer has a high rate of response ($\geq 50\%$) to combination cytotoxic therapy, especially regimens that are designed around cisplatin. Approximately 50% of patients with high-grade bladder cancer and deep muscle invasion ultimately die of disseminated disease. High-risk patients with pT3–pT4 and node-negative disease have no more than a 5-year overall survival of 47% after cystectomy; patients with lymph node metastases have an overall 5-year survival rate of up to 31% after radical cystectomy [1,2]. However, translating the high response seen in locally advanced disease into long-term survival in the metastatic setting and to improved survival in the advanced setting has proved difficult [3,4]. This article reviews the use of adjuvant chemotherapy in localized or locally advanced transitional cell cancer. The chemotherapy of urological malignancies, including bladder cancer, has recently been reviewed in detail [5]; this article does not contain an extensive review of the drugs used.

Role of systemic therapy in urothelial cancer: regimen selection

Cisplatin has been the cornerstone of systemic therapy for advanced urothelial cancer for 25 years and remains so (Table 1) [6–21]. Table 2

details the acronyms, schedule, and dosing of more commonly used chemotherapy regimens for urothelial cancer [20,22–25]. Sequential trials in this setting tell us that: cisplatin is superior to supportive care, at least in contemporaneous controls; combination therapy with methotrexate, vinblastine, doxorubicin, and cisplatin (MVAC) is superior to cisplatin alone [14] and to cyclophosphamide, doxorubicin, and cisplatin (CISCA) [15]; and therapy with gemcitabine and cisplatin is equivalent to MVAC but has less morbidity [20]. Several other platin-based combinations have shown promising activity in phase II trials, including ifosfamide, paclitaxel, and cisplatin and cisplatin or carboplatin, gemcitabine, and a taxane [23,25–27]. Whether triplet therapy carries any advantage over doublet therapy has yet to be demonstrated. The European Organization for the Research and Treatment of Cancer (EORTC) with the assistance of the Southwest Oncology Group (SWOG) and several other groups have concluded a trial comparing gemcitabine and cisplatin (GC) with GC plus paclitaxel in advanced transitional cell cancer (TCC) with results available soon [21]. Carboplatin is a popular alternative to cisplatin in some centers, but its equivalence to cisplatin has not be shown in transitional cell carcinoma and its use should probably be reserved for patients with impaired renal function or other contraindication to cisplatin except in the context of a clinical trial [28].

In terms of duration of therapy for advanced transitional cancer, most clinicians do not continue therapy indefinitely until progression or extreme

---

* Corresponding author.

E-mail address: quinn_d@ccnt.hsc.usc.edu
(D.I. Quinn).

Table 1
A brief history of systemic chemotherapy for metastatic
transitional cell cancer

Year	Advance made	References
1976	Cisplatin enters clinical trials and demonstrates single agent activity in TCC as does doxorubicin	[6–8]
1981–1982	Methotrexate and vinblastine demonstrate single agent activity in TCC	[9,10]
1985	MVAC and CMV combinations reported	[11–13]
1990–1992	MVAC demonstrated superior to cisplatin alone and cisplatin, cyclophosphamide, doxorubicin in combination	[14–16]
1993	Taxanes demonstrates single agent activity in TCC Ifosfamide "active" in TCC	[17,18]
1996	Gemcitabine demonstrates single agent activity in TCC	[19]
2000	Gemcitabine and cisplatin equivalent in efficacy to MVAC with less toxicity	[20]
2004	EORTC trial of GC versus GC plus paclitaxel completed	[21]

Abbreviations: CMV, cisplatin, methotrexate, and
vinblastine; EORTC, European Organization for the
Research and Treatment of Cancer; GC, gemcitabine
and cisplatin; MVAC, methotrexate, vinblastine, doxorubicin, and cisplatin; TCC, transitional cell cancer.

toxicity. Rather, a defined course of therapy is given
until maximal response is assessed to be achieved.
While there is little definitive evidence for this,
experience in non–small cell lung cancer and breast
cancer suggests that this response is generally
obtained in the first 9 weeks of therapy and further
response is unlikely after 12 to 18 weeks and
certainly after 24 weeks.

A historical review of the clinical trials of adjuvant chemotherapy

Multiple cisplatin-based combinations have
been evaluated in the adjuvant setting after the
promising results of cisplatin-based therapy for
patients with metastatic disease (Table 3) [29–37].
Logothetis and colleagues [38] administered

CISCA to a group of 71 postcystectomy patients
with resected nodal metastases, extravesicular
extension, lymphovascular invasion, or pelvic
visceral invasion. These patients were compared
in a nonrandomized fashion with 62 high-risk
patients and 206 low-risk patients who did not
receive adjuvant chemotherapy. The authors concluded that adjuvant CISCA conferred a 2-year
disease-free survival advantage to patients with
unfavorable pathologic findings (70% vs 30%;
$P = .00012$). The earliest randomized control trial
of combination chemotherapy administered to
patients after radical cystectomy was conducted
at the University of Southern California (USC)
[39]. Ninety-one patients with p3, p4, or node-
positive TCC were randomized to four cycles of
cyclophosphamide, adriamycin (doxorubicin), cisplatin (CAP) or to observation. Chemotherapy
resulted in a significant improvement in the risk of
disease recurrence at 3 years (0.30 vs 0.54;
$P = .011$ [unstratified Wilcoxon test]) and in the
overall risk of death (0.34 vs 0.50; $P = .099$
[unstratified Wilcoxon]). The median survival of
patients on chemotherapy was reported to be 4.25
years versus 2.4 years for patients in the observation group. This study has been criticized for the
fact that only 33 out of 44 patients assigned to the
chemotherapy arm received one or more cycles of
CAP, for the small sample size, and for deficien-
cies in statistical analysis such as the use of the
Wilcoxon test emphasizing early differences.
Nonetheless, the study was provocative in re-
vealing the potential benefit of adjuvant chemotherapy and in highlighting the difficulties
involved in conducting such trials.

A subsequent trial of adjuvant chemotherapy
with three cycles of cisplatin alone did not result
in any survival benefit in a randomized study of 77
patients [40]. Potential explanations for the lack of
significant benefit include the use of single-agent
cisplatin, the small sample size, the inclusion of
patients with lower T stage and lymph node–
negative disease, and the administration of the
three planned cycles of chemotherapy to only
65% of patients in the treatment arm.

Given the superiority of the MVAC combination over single-agent cisplatin in the metastatic
setting [14], it became important to evaluate the
MVAC or methotrexate, vinblastine, epirubicin,
and cisplatin (MVEC) combinations in the adjuvant setting. Stockle and colleagues [41] randomized patients with pT3, pT4, and/or pelvic lymph
nodes to three cycles of MVAC or MVEC versus
observation. Although the study intended to accrue

Table 2
Commonly used combination chemotherapy regimens

Abbreviation	Drugs used	Cycle duration	Schedule	Reference
MVAC	Methotrexate	4 weeks	Days 1, 15, 22	[20,22]
	Vinblastine		Days 1, 15, 22	
	Doxorubicin		Day 2	
	Cisplatin		Day 2	
GC	Cisplatin	4 weeks	70 mg/m^2 day 1	[20]
	Gemcitabine		1000 mg/m^2 days 1, 8, 15	
GC	Cisplatin	3 weeks	37.5 mg/m^2 day 1, 2	Unpublished University
	Gemcitabine		1000 mg/m^2 day 1, 8	of Southern California
				in-house regimen
ITP	Ifosfamide	3 weeks	1.5 g/m^2 days 1, 2, 3	[23,24]
	Paclitaxel		200 mg/m^2 day 1	
	Cisplatin		70 mg/m^2 day 1	
AG-TP	Doxorubicin	2 weeks (×4)	50 mg/m^2	Unpublished MSKCC
	Gemcitabine		2000 mg/m^2	97-106, used in
	then			CALGB 90104
	Paclitaxel	2 weeks (×4)	150 mg/m^2	
	Cisplatin		60 mg/m^2	
GTC	Paclitaxel	3 weeks	200 mg/m^2 day 1	[24,25]
	Gemcitabine		800 mg/m^2 days 1, 8	
	Carboplatin		Area under the concentration	
			curve (estimated) = 5*	
GCT	Gemcitabine	3 weeks	800 mg/m^2 days 1, 8	[24]
	Cisplatin		70 mg/m^2 day 2	
	Paclitaxel		200 mg/m^2 day 1	

Abbreviations: CALGB, Cancer and Leukemia Group B; MSKCC, Memorial Sloan Kettering Cancer Center.
(*Data from* Calvert AH, Newell DR, Gumbrell LA, et al. Carboplatin dosage: prospective evaluation of a simple formula based on renal function. J Clin Oncol 1989;7:1748–56.)

100 patients, it was closed after an interim analysis of 49 randomized patients revealed a significant advantage in relapse-free survival with chemotherapy (P = .0015). This trial has been interpreted with caution given its early closure and the fact that only 62% of patients randomized to chemotherapy completed the three cycles of treatment. Furthermore, patients in the observation arm were not offered at relapse. Three years later, the same authors reported their longer experience with adjuvant MVAC/MVEC in 83 patients [30]. Forty-nine of the patients had been enrolled in the prospective trial before being closed, while the remaining 38 had received MVAC/MVEC as a routinely recommended therapy based on the interim results of the trial. Longer follow-up of the patients (38 to 78 months) who were on the trial continued to reveal a significant improvement in progression-free survival in the adjuvant chemotherapy group (P = .0005). The continued advantage in progression-free survival with more mature data offered support to the beneficial role of chemotherapy.

The combination of cisplatin, vinblastine, and methotrexate was used as adjuvant therapy in a prospective randomized trial of four cycles of cisplatin, methotrexate, and vinblastine versus observation following cystectomy at Stanford [33]. Patients accrued to this trial had p3b and p4 TCC with or without lymph node involvement. Data were reported on 50 out of 55 enrolled patients; 22 out of 25 patients randomized to adjuvant therapy received the total number of four planned cycles. With a median follow-up of 62 months, a significant difference in freedom from progression was noted between the chemotherapy and the observation group (median of 37 months vs. 12 months, respectively; P = .01). No significant difference in overall survival was noted.

Adjuvant and other adjunctive chemotherapeutic approaches

The administration of chemotherapy for localized bladder cancer can in the setting of neoadjuvant, concurrent or adjuvant therapy (see Table 3). Each has its advantages and clinical proponents. Neoadjuvant therapy allows us to see whether the cancer responds and allows the patient

Table 3
Summary of key studies of adjuvant and neoadjuvant chemotherapy in bladder cancer

Center	Regimen	Outcome	Comment	Reference
Adjuvant				
University of Mainz	MVEC/MVAC	Early stopping because of interim analysis favoring chemotherapy	Underpowered	[30]
University of Southern California	Cisplatin-based	Modest benefit for chemotherapy	Methodologic issues	[1,31]
Stanford University	CMV	Early stopping because of interim analysis favoring chemotherapy	Underpowered, delayed time to progression ($P = .01$) effect on survival	[32]
Neoadjuvant				
MRC/EORTC	CMV	Absolute improvement in survival of 5.5% ($P = .075$)		[33]
RTOG	Radiation therapy with cisplatin with or without adjuvant CMV	No difference in PFS or OS		[34]
Nordic trials I and II	Cisplatin/ doxorubicin and cisplatin/ methotrexate	OS 56 vs 48% at 5 years favored chemotherapy ($P = .04$)		[35,36]
SWOG Intergroup 8710	MVAC	OS favored chemotherapy	P_0 patients after chemotherapy had a very good outcome	[37]

Abbreviations: CMV, cisplatin, methotrexate, and vinblastine; MRC, Medical Research Council; MVEC, methotrexate, vinblastine, epirubicin, and cisplatin; OS, Overall survival; PFS, Progression-free survival; RTOG, Radiation Therapy Oncology Group.

to experience chemotherapy in the absence of postoperative morbidity. Adjuvant therapy, in a postoperative context, allows us to give treatment based on a very accurate concept of the disease stage. A single study has compared the two approaches and found outcomes to be very similar for patients with transitional cell carcinoma [42,43]. One exception to this is with a diagnosis of small cell or neuroendocrine bladder cancer in which neoadjuvant therapy with platin and etoposide produces a markedly improved survival rate based on data from M.D. Anderson Cancer Center [44] and a similar experience at USC. Based on these data, M.D. Anderson Cancer Center have an ongoing neoadjuvant study with a combination of four cytotoxic agents followed by surgery in nonmetastatic small cell bladder cancer.

In an effort to improve outcome for patients with locally advanced disease, a number of trials of neoadjuvant and adjuvant therapy have been undertaken or are ongoing (Tables 3 and 4) [30–38,45–48]. Generally, the outcome of these trials

in terms of survival have been of a modest to statistically borderline benefit in favor of chemotherapy. Some of these studies have demonstrated a statistically significant advantage to either adjuvant or neoadjuvant therapy [21,31,34,38, 49,50]. The SWOG study of neoadjuvant MVAC as well as the Nordic trials suggest a modest survival benefit from neoadjuvant chemotherapy. Of note in the SWOG trial was that patients who had no detectable disease at cystectomy had a very good prognosis compared with those with any residual disease. In a recent European study, MVAC chemotherapy was given to 109 patients with clinical stage T2-T4, N0, M0 transitional cell bladder cancer, with 49% of patients having no residual disease at cystoscopy. These patients were given the option of further therapy, including cystectomy or radiation therapy, or observation with a 5-year overall survival in excess of 70%. This suggests that chemotherapy response is a good predictor of subsequent disease-free and overall survival and may allow some patients to be

Table 4
Summary of ongoing and recently completed studies of adjuvant chemotherapy after radical cystectomy for bladder cancer

Center	Regimen	Outcome	Comment	Reference
CALGB 90104	AG-TP vs GC	Ongoing	T3, T4, or N+	[45]
EORTC 30994	Postoperative vs delayed chemotherapy (MVAC or GC)	Ongoing	T3, T4, or N+	[45]
SWOG	MVAC vs no chemotherapy	Ongoing	T1, T2a, T2b N0 P53 (+) by IHC	[45,46]
NCI, Cairo University, Egypt	XRT vs XRT + GC	Ongoing 59 points accrued to date	High proportion of squamous cell carcinoma	[47]
Multicenter, Germany	CM vs MVEC	N = 324 Progression-free survival equivalent in both arms	Grade III/IV leukopenia 22% in MVEC arm vs 6% in CM arm Two study related-deaths in CM arm	[48]
Ospedale S. Maria, Annunziata, Italy	GC	Phase II N = 40	Grade III/IV hematologic toxicities in 10% of patients	[48]

Abbreviations: CALGB, Cancer and Leukemia Group B; CM, Cisplatin-Methotrexate; IHC, Immunohistochemistry; NCI, National Cancer Institute; RT, Radiation therapy.

observed without radiation or surgery [51]. However, clear and clinically irrefutable benefit is yet to be demonstrated for adjuvant therapy and is the focus of a currently accruing EORTC trial of adjuvant GC compared with the same regimen if and when disease recrudescence occurs [21]. Two recent meta-analyses reemphasize the concept of a small benefit in favor of neoadjuvant or adjuvant chemotherapy, particularly for regimens incorporating cisplatin [52,53].

Approach to cystectomy in patients who have a high risk of postoperative relapse and death

Patients have their risk of relapse defined by pathologic staging at surgery. At USC and many other American institutions, patients with pT3, pT4, or N+ disease are referred for medical oncology consultation. Several issues must be addressed so that the patient can make an informed decision regarding adjuvant chemotherapy. These include:

• the patient's estimated risk of relapse based on the untreated natural history of the patient's disease
• the conceptual basis of adjuvant therapy in attempting to eradicate residual cancer cells

while they are at their lowest concentration in the body
• the success of adjuvant chemotherapy in improving survival in patients with locally advanced breast, colorectal, or lung cancer
• the high response rates obtained in the treatment of metastatic urothelial cancer contrasted with the low cure rate in that setting
• the relatively modest effect of chemotherapy in improving disease-free and overall survival in studies of patients with high-risk urothelial cancer; we quote a 5% to 15% absolute improvement in 5-year survival based on USC and published experiences
• the choice of chemotherapy:
    MVAC versus more recently derived combinations incorporating gemcitabine, such as GC
    Equivalence for efficacy with a better toxicity profile for GC over MVAC in metastatic-stage TCC
    Lack of comparative data on MVAC versus other regimens in the adjuvant setting

For the patient, the decision-making process is complex. Patients considering adjuvant chemotherapy entertain factors including the relative risk for their disease (lymph node involvement or not), geographical proximity to the treatment center, and the toxicity of the regimens offered relative to the absolute potential benefit. From the perspective of the oncologist, the factors involved include the age and performance status of the patient and comorbid conditions, especially renal and cardiac function. In our practice, 90% of patients elect for adjuvant therapy, and approximately 65% of patients opt for GC rather than MVAC. Most patients who receive MVAC are less than 65 years of age and have excellent performance status and normal renal function.

Specific challenges in administration of chemotherapy: managing in the face of premorbid conditions and toxicities

All patients are offered 12 weeks of therapy: three cycles of 28-day MVAC or four cycles of GC given over a 21-day period. Therapy should commence 6–12 weeks after surgery for an adjuvant effect. We generally like to see the patient eat normally and gain weight after surgery before commencing chemotherapy. Our institutional policy for cisplatin administration is for the dose to be split over two successive days with a full liter of intravenous hydration fluid before and after each dose of cisplatin. Diuretics are not given unless the patient manifests clinical fluid overload. We provide antiemetic support for acute and delay nausea and vomiting with a 5HT3 antagonist and dexamethasone therapy as per standard antiemetic guidelines [54,55]. Oral dexamethasone is continued at a dose of 4 mg each morning on days 3 through 7 as a prophylaxis while as-needed oral metoclopramide or prochlorperazine is prescribed [56]. In certain patients, adjunctive targeting of the γ-aminobutyric acid ionophore with benzodiazepines such as lorazepam can be useful in controlling acute nausea. Patients who are at high risk for nausea and vomiting based on predefined factors (female, lifelong nonsmokers, nonethanol users, prior hyperemesis of pregnancy or motion sickness, or prior uncontrolled chemotherapy-induced nausea and vomiting) are also offered a neurokinin-1 inhibitor such as aprepitant [57].

Renal impairment

Patients with renal impairment of any level are generally not offered MVAC because of issues with renal clearance of methotrexate and toxicity from cisplatin; however, they may be considered for therapy with GC. In patients with a serum creatinine level up to 2 mg/dL or a creatinine clearance of 50 mL·kg·min, we do not modify cisplatin administration, although the incidence of cytopenias is increased in patients who have renal impairment and may require a dose reduction in gemcitabine. We do not offer adjuvant therapy incorporating carboplatin in renally impaired patients because of a lack of evidence for benefit. If the patient has a creatinine level of more than 2 mg/mL (170 μmol/L) or a creatinine clearance below 50 mL/min, then we would recommend close observation rather than adjuvant therapy.

Left ventricular impairment

In patients who have any degree of symptomatic heart failure (New York Heart Association grade 2 or above) or an estimated left ventricular ejection fraction of less than 45% on nucleotide cardiac scan or echocardiography should not receive doxorubicin and therefore are not candidates for MVAC. These patients may also have problems tolerating the fluid loading required for cisplatin but can be managed with judicious use of diuretics for clinical fluid overload in most cases.

Mucositis (typically evidenced by mouth ulcers) can be troublesome, especially around day 15 of the MVAC protocol. This is best treated with regular mouthwashes of weak saline or bicarbonate solution supplemented with oral antifungal therapy such as nystatin. Ongoing mucositis for more than 72 hours or that associated with pain on swallowing should raise concern regarding oro-esophageal candidiasis, which requires therapy with ingested or injected systemic antifungal therapy, typically fluconazole. Severe mucositis can manifest as abdominal pain and diarrhea. The combination of mucositis or diarrhea and neutropenia with or without fever can be potentially lethal and can occasionally require rapid treatment in an inpatient facility.

Cytopenias

Neutropenic and thrombocytopenia are common effects of cytotoxic chemotherapy. Most patients experience these transiently and asymptomatically during their therapy and never require intervention. However, a smaller number of patients develop systemic symptoms of infection during neutropenia, including fever, chills, rigors, or unexplained lethargy. These patients need to be aggressively treated with antibiotics that cover gram-negative bacilli such as *Pseudomonas* and

Klebsiella species, which untreated can be rapidly fatal. The development of oral fluoroquinolones that encompass such coverage have moved the therapy of febrile neutropenia in otherwise well patients into the outpatient setting. Patients who have indwelling intravenous devices also require coverage of gram-positive organisms if presenting with febrile neutropenia. More rarely, fungal septicemia can be a problem, especially in patients treated with prolonged broad spectrum antibiotics in the perioperative period or with underlying diabetes mellitus. Thrombocytopenia can lead to unusual bleeding, particularly from the nose or gastrointestinal tract or at the site of trauma. Patients who have significant bleeding or have a platelet count of less then 20,000 per microliter should receive a platelet transfusion. We do not routinely use erythropoietin, granulocyte–colony-stimulating factors, or thrombopoietin in our patients who receive chemotherapy because of a lack of demonstrated benefit for most patients coupled with considerable cost. However, in response to specific problems seen in early cycles of chemotherapy, subsequent cycles may incorporate these agents when indicated [58].

New cisplatin-based combinations in the adjuvant setting

Taxanes and gemcitabine have been used in different combinations with cisplatin to treat metastatic bladder TCC. The combination of GC has similar survival outcomes with less toxicity compared with MVAC in the metastatic setting [20]. Recent data support the safety and feasibility of this regimen when administered as adjuvant therapy after cystectomy [59,60]. The most significant toxicity in both series was hematologic with thrombocytopenia and neutropenia in up to 50% of patients. We recently presented part of our experience with adjuvant GC in a group of 25 patients with pT3 and pT4 disease with or without lymph node involvement. A similar incidence of hematologic toxicity was noted with only 2 out of 25 patients having grade 3 nonhematologic toxicity. At a median follow-up of 27.7 months, the median time to recurrence was 43 months and the median survival was 54.2+ months [61]. This compares favorably to the historically reported median survival of 51 months with adjuvant cyclophosphamide, doxorubicin, and cisplatin and 63 months with cisplatin, methotrexate, and vinblastine. Our report in combination with the safety and feasibility data reported by other investigators suggests that

GC is a promising combination with a favorable toxicity profile that deserves further evaluation in a prospective randomized trial. The EORTC is conducting an international trial of chemotherapy after cystectomy versus chemotherapy at the time of relapse, with GC being one of the regimens available to investigators.

The Hellenic Cooperative Oncology Group evaluated the combination of paclitaxel and carboplatin in a group of 92 patients. The baseline characteristics of the patients were comparable to our series (pT3 or greater or with lymph node involvement), but 26% of them did not undergo a lymphadenectomy, and 15% had nontransitional cell histology. At a median follow-up of 36.6 months, they estimated a 5-year overall survival of 28.9%, which is probably inferior to historical controls. Grade 3 or 4 toxicity was mostly hematologic, with 17 cases (19%) of neutropenia. Four patients only had grade 3 or 4 nonhematologic toxicity. There were two deaths, possibly related to chemotherapy [62]. These data do not encourage the use of this regimen in the adjuvant setting, especially given the inferiority of this combination to the cisplatin-containing standard in advanced disease [28]. However, the incorporation of taxanes and other active agents into adjuvant trials is important and justified given the poor outcome in the subset of patients with locally advanced disease. The Cancer and Leukemia Group B recently launched a trial comparing GC and an alternating second weekly "dose dense" regimen of doxorubicin with gemcitabine and paclitaxel with cisplatin (see Tables 2 and 4 and http://www.ctsu.org). Although this study will not incorporate a control arm of no therapy nor of MVAC, it will address issues regarding the comparative efficacy and tolerability of these regimens in this group of patients. It will also explore the value of putative tissue markers of efficacy and outcome to determine whether patients can be preselected for one regimen or the other.

Multimodal approaches incorporating radiation therapy

Although the focus of this article is on adjuvant chemotherapy therapy after cystectomy, a discussion of chemotherapy and radiation is warranted to encompass the issues of neoadjuvant radiation therapy before cystectomy and the key role of salvage cystectomy in patients offered primary chemoradiation therapy for their localized bladder cancer.

A retrospective study undertaken at USC for patients treated between 1971 and 1982 suggested no disease control or mortality benefit to 4 fraction of preoperative radiation therapy to a dose of 1600 cGy compared with cystectomy alone [63]. While not constituting a prospective, randomized evaluation of the question of an advantage of neo-adjuvant radiation treatment in this setting, this study diminished enthusiasm for this approach. Other groups working contemporaneously examined the role of "sandwich" radiation or adjuvant radiation in the perioperative period [64,65]. Although these studies suggested a potential improvement in local disease control, particularly in cases with pT3B, pT4, or margin positive disease, the consequent toxicity especially visited upon the gastrointestinal tract dissuaded routine use or further prospective evaluation [64–66]. As a result, neither pre- nor postoperative radiation therapy is routinely employed as an adjunct to cystectomy for transitional cell carcinoma.

Most chemotherapy regimens used in combination with radiation for bladder cancer have been designed around cisplatin. The general paradigm has been to treat with radiation and concurrent weekly intravenous cisplatin with a review for response at 4000 cGy [35,67–69]. Patients not responding may then be offered salvage surgery, because their outcome is decidedly poor in the absence of this. Patients responding and proceeding to full doses (of the order of 6500 cGy) of radiation therapy with chemotherapy have similar recurrence and survival risks to those treated with cystoprostatectomy while maintaining their bladder and in most cases having their bladder function preserved [70]. Studies to determine whether the addition of a multiple drug regimen before or after concurrent cisplatin and radiation therapy have failed to demonstrate a benefit in local control, time to progression, or overall survival [67]. Eapen and colleagues [71] have experimented with intra-arterial cisplatin concurrent with radiation therapy for localized bladder cancer and impressive response and cancer control rates. However, the use of this approach will require randomized trials comparing intra-arterial and intravenous therapy.

Molecular markers of outcome, the efficacy of systemic therapy, and potential of targeted therapeutics

Molecular markers have value in defining the natural history of localized bladder cancer treated surgically [72]. Abnormalities of p53, p21, and retinoblastoma protein can predict survival following cystectomy [73–76]. A currently accruing trial predicated on the p53 status of patients with pT2 disease aims to test the effect of three cycles of adjuvant MVAC chemotherapy in this population and should provide data on the potential interaction between these molecular factors and cytotoxic chemotherapy [46].

Response prediction based on tissue markers has been a long-term aim of many scientific investigators and commercial interests. It is important to note that none of the recently available methods pass stringency standards to allow recommendation for use in a clinical setting [77]. However, several new markers of chemotherapy intracellular trafficking or target integrity are being evaluated for response predictions across a range of tumors in prospective clinical trials. Among the most promising of these are nucleotide

Table 5
Newer agents targeting specific molecules in bladder cancer

Target	Agents	References
Tubulins	Taxanes, epothilones, CT-2103	[96,97]
Kinetic spindle protein	SB-715992	[98]
DNA cross links: novel platinums	Oxaliplatin	[80,99]
Topoisomerase I	Irinotecan, topotecan	[100,101]
Cyclooxygenase 2	Celecoxib	[102,103]
Epidermal growth factor receptor family	EGFr: cetuximab, gefitinib, erlotinib	[104–106]
	Her2/neu: trastuzumab	[105,107]
Blood vessels	VEGF: bevacizumab, VEGF Trap, veglin	[108–111]
	VEGFR2: SU11248, PTK787, BAY 43-9006	[112–116]
	Thrombospondin mimetics: ABT-510	[117–118]
Proteosome	Bortezomib	[119–121]
Histone deacetylase	Depsipeptide, SAHA	[122–126]

Abbreviations: EGF, epidermal growth factor receptor; SAHA, suberoylanilide hydroxamic acid; VEGF, vascular endothelial growth factor.

excision repair pathway molecules such as ERCC1 (excision repair cross complementation group 1) [78–84]. Low expression of ERCC1 predicts improved response to and outcome from platinum-based therapy in several malignancies, including ovarian [85,86], colorectal [87], esophageal [88], gastric [89], and non–small cell lung cancers [90]. High expression is also linked to resistance to radiation therapy in a number of model systems [91–93]. Targeting of this pathway with response modulators may increase sensitivity to platinum compounds in patients with high levels of nucleotide excision repair pathway molecules and who, on this basis, would normally be chemo- and radio-resistant [94,95].

In the era of molecular targeted therapies, single-agent trials of these agents have to date been disappointing in bladder cancer as with many other cancers. Bladder cancers often have an aberrance of epidermal growth factor, Her2/neu, and vascular endothelial growth pathways. The modulation of these pathways as well as epigenetic processes such as proteosome activity and methylation status may yield much therapeutic profit, either alone or in combination with cytotoxic and radiation therapy (Table 5) [96–126]. The challenge is to design clinical trials that test these combinations in a rigorous but safe environment [127].

References

[1] Stein JP, Lieskovsky G, Cote R, et al. Radical cystectomy in the treatment of invasive bladder cancer: long-term results in 1,054 patients. J Clin Oncol 2001;19:666–75.

[2] Frank I, Cheville JC, Blute ML, et al. Transitional cell carcinoma of the urinary bladder with regional lymph node involvement treated by cystectomy: clinicopathologic features associated with outcome. Cancer 2003;97:2425–31.

[3] Igawa M, Urakami S, Shiina H, Ishibe T, Kadena H, Usui T. Long-term results with M-VAC for advanced urothelial cancer: high relapse rate and low survival in patients with a complete response. Br J Urol 1995;76:321–4.

[4] Juffs HG, Moore MJ, Tannock IF. The role of systemic chemotherapy in the management of muscle-invasive bladder cancer. Lancet Oncol 2002;3: 738–47.

[5] Quinn DI, Creaven PJ, Raghavan D. Principles of chemotherapy for genitourinary cancer. In: Richie JP, D'Amico AV, editors. Urologica oncology. Philadephia: Elsevier; 2005. p. 57–81.

[6] Burchenal JH, Kalaher K, Dew K, et al. Rationale for development of platinum analogs. Cancer Treat Rep 1979;63:1493–8.

[7] Yagoda A. Phase II trials with cis-dichlorodiammineplatinum(II) in the treatment of urothelial cancer. Cancer Treat Rep 1979;63:1565–72.

[8] Weinstein SH, Schmidt JD. Doxorubicin chemotherapy in advanced transitional cell carcinoma. Urology 1976;8:336–41.

[9] Natale RB, Yagoda A, Watson RC, et al. Methotrexate: an active drug in bladder cancer. Cancer 1981;47:1246–50.

[10] Blumenreich MS, Yagoda A, Natale RB, et al. Phase II trial of vinblastine sulfate for metastatic urothelial tract tumors. Cancer 1982;50:435–8.

[11] Harker WG, Meyers FJ, Freiha FS, et al. Cisplatin, methotrexate, and vinblastine (CMV): an effective chemotherapy regimen for metastatic transitional cell carcinoma of the urinary tract. A Northern California Oncology Group study. J Clin Oncol 1985;3:1463–70.

[12] Sternberg CN, Yagoda A, Scher HI, et al. Preliminary results of M-VAC (methotrexate, vinblastine, doxorubicin and cisplatin) for transitional cell carcinoma of the urothelium. J Urol 1985;133:403–7.

[13] Sternberg CN, Yagoda A, Scher HI, et al. M-VAC (methotrexate, vinblastine, doxorubicin and cisplatin) for advanced transitional cell carcinoma of the urothelium. J Urol 1988;139:461–9.

[14] Loehrer Sr PJ, Einhorn LH, Elson PJ, et al. A randomized comparison of cisplatin alone or in combination with methotrexate, vinblastine, and doxorubicin in patients with metastatic urothelial carcinoma: a cooperative group study. J Clin Oncol 1992;10:1066–73.

[15] Logothetis CJ, Dexeus FH, Finn L, et al. A prospective randomized trial comparing MVAC and CISCA chemotherapy for patients with metastatic urothelial tumors. J Clin Oncol 1990;8:1050–5.

[16] Saxman SB, Propert KJ, Einhorn LH, et al. Long-term follow-up of a phase III intergroup study of cisplatin alone or in combination with methotrexate, vinblastine, and doxorubicin in patients with metastatic urothelial carcinoma: a cooperative group study. J Clin Oncol 1997;15:2564–9.

[17] Roth BJ, Dreicer R, Einhorn LH, et al. Significant activity of paclitaxel in advanced transitional-cell carcinoma of the urothelium: a phase II trial of the Eastern Cooperative Oncology Group. J Clin Oncol 1994;12:2264–70.

[18] Roth BJ. Ifosfamide in the treatment of bladder cancer. Semin Oncol 1996;23(Suppl 6):50–5.

[19] Stadler WM, Kuzel T, Roth B, et al. Phase II study of single-agent gemcitabine in previously untreated patients with metastatic urothelial cancer. J Clin Oncol 1997;15:3394–8.

[20] von der Maase H, Hansen SW, Roberts JT, et al. Gemcitabine and cisplatin versus methotrexate, vinblastine, doxorubicin, and cisplatin in advanced or metastatic bladder cancer: results of a large, randomized, multinational, multicenter, phase III study. J Clin Oncol 2000;18:3068–77.

[21] De Wit R. Overview of bladder cancer trials in the European Organization for Research and Treatment. Cancer 2003;97:2120–6.

[22] Dodd PM, McCaffrey JA, Herr H, et al. Outcome of postchemotherapy surgery after treatment with methotrexate, vinblastine, doxorubicin, and cisplatin in patients with unresectable or metastatic transitional cell carcinoma. J Clin Oncol 1999;17:2546–52.

[23] Bajorin DF, McCaffrey JA, Dodd PM, et al. Ifosfamide, paclitaxel, and cisplatin for patients with advanced transitional cell carcinoma of the urothelial tract: final report of a phase II trial evaluating two dosing schedules. Cancer 2000;88:1671–8.

[24] de Wit R, Bellmunt J. Overview of gemcitabine triplets in metastatic bladder cancer. Crit Rev Oncol Hematol 2003;45:191–7.

[25] Hussain M, Vaishampayan U, Smith DC. Novel gemcitabine-containing triplets in the management of urothelial cancer. Semin Oncol 2002;29:20–4.

[26] Bajorin DF, McCaffrey JA, Hilton S, et al. Treatment of patients with transitional-cell carcinoma of the urothelial tract with ifosfamide, paclitaxel, and cisplatin: a phase II trial. J Clin Oncol 1998;16:2722–7.

[27] Hussain M, Vaishampayan U, Du W, Redman B, Smith DC. Combination paclitaxel, carboplatin, and gemcitabine is an active treatment for advanced urothelial cancer. J Clin Oncol 2001;19:2527–33.

[28] Dreicer R, Manola J, Roth BJ, et al. Phase III trial of methotrexate, vinblastine, doxorubicin, and cisplatin versus carboplatin and paclitaxel in patients with advanced carcinoma of the urothelium. Cancer 2004;100:1639–45.

[29] Hussain SA, James ND. The systemic treatment of advanced and metastatic bladder cancer. Lancet Oncol 2003;4:489–97.

[30] Stockle M, Meyenburg W, Wellek S, et al. Adjuvant polychemotherapy of nonorgan-confined bladder cancer after radical cystectomy revisited: long-term results of a controlled prospective study and further clinical experience. J Urol 1995;153:47–52.

[31] Skinner DG, Daniels JR, Russell CA, et al. The role of adjuvant chemotherapy following cystectomy for invasive bladder cancer: a prospective comparative trial. J Urol 1991;145:459–64 [discussion: 464–7].

[32] Freiha F, Reese J, Torti FM. A randomized trial of radical cystectomy versus radical cystectomy plus cisplatin, vinblastine and methotrexate chemotherapy for muscle invasive bladder cancer. J Urol 1996;155:495–9 [discussion: 499–500].

[33] Medical Research Council. Neoadjuvant cisplatin, methotrexate, and vinblastine chemotherapy for muscle-invasive bladder cancer: a randomised controlled trial. International collaboration of trialists. Lancet 1999;354:533–40.

[34] Shipley WU, Winter KA, Kaufman DS, et al. Phase III trial of neoadjuvant chemotherapy in patients with invasive bladder cancer treated with selective bladder preservation by combined radiation therapy and chemotherapy: initial results of Radiation Therapy Oncology Group 89–03. J Clin Oncol 1998;16:3576–83.

[35] Malmstrom PU, Rintala E, Wahlqvist R, et al. Five-year followup of a prospective trial of radical cystectomy and neoadjuvant chemotherapy: Nordic Cystectomy Trial I. The Nordic Cooperative Bladder Cancer Study Group. J Urol 1996;155:1903–6.

[36] Sherif A, Holmberg L, Rintala E, et al. Neoadjuvant cisplatinum based combination chemotherapy in patients with invasive bladder cancer: a combined analysis of two Nordic studies. Eur Urol 2004;45:297–303.

[37] Grossman HB, Natale RB, Tangen CM, et al. Neoadjuvant chemotherapy plus cystectomy compared with cystectomy alone for locally advanced bladder cancer. N Engl J Med 2003;349:859–66.

[38] Logothetis CJ, Johnson DE, Chong C, et al. Adjuvant cyclophosphamide, doxorubicin, and cisplatin chemotherapy for bladder cancer: an update. J Clin Oncol 1988;6:1590–6.

[39] Skinner DG, Daniels JR, Lieskovsky G. Current status of adjuvant chemotherapy after radical cystectomy for deeply invasive bladder cancer. Urology 1984;24:46–52.

[40] Studer UE, Bacchi M, Biedermann C, et al. Adjuvant cisplatin chemotherapy following cystectomy for bladder cancer: results of a prospective randomized trial. J Urol 1994;152:81–4.

[41] Stockle M, Meyenburg W, Wellek S, et al. Advanced bladder cancer (stages pT3b, pT4a, pN1 and pN2): improved survival after radical cystectomy and 3 adjuvant cycles of chemotherapy. Results of a controlled prospective study. J Urol 1992;148:302–6 [discussion: 306–7].

[42] Logothetis C, Swanson D, Amato R, et al. Optimal delivery of perioperative chemotherapy: preliminary results of a randomized, prospective, comparative trial of preoperative and postoperative chemotherapy for invasive bladder carcinoma. J Urol 1996;155:1241–5.

[43] Millikan R, Dinney C, Swanson D, et al. Integrated therapy for locally advanced bladder cancer: final report of a randomized trial of cystectomy plus adjuvant M-VAC versus cystectomy with both preoperative and postoperative M-VAC. J Clin Oncol 2001;19:4005–13.

[44] Siefker-Radtke AO, Dinney CP, Abrahams NA, et al. Evidence supporting preoperative chemotherapy for small cell carcinoma of the bladder: a retrospective review of the M.D. Anderson cancer experience. J Urol 2004;172:481–4.

[45] Garcia JA, Dreicer R. Adjuvant and neoadjuvant chemotherapy for bladder cancer: management

and controversies. Nature Clinical Practice. Urology 2005;2:32–7.

[46] Crawford ED, Wood DP, Petrylak DP, et al. Southwest Oncology Group studies in bladder cancer. Cancer 2003;97(Suppl):2099–108.

[47] Zaghloul MS, Khaled H, Lotyef M, et al. Adjuvant chemoradiotherapy with gemcitabine and cisplatin and postoperative radiotherapy (PORT) versus PORT alone in high risk bladder cancer patients. A phase III randomized controlled trial. ASCO Annual Meeting Proceedings, New Orleans, LA. Journal of Clinical Oncology 2004;22(Suppl):4626.

[48] Lehmann J, Retz M, Weining C, et al. Adjuvant cisplatin, methotrexate (CM) versus methotrexate, vinblastine, epirubicin and cisplatin (MVEC) for locally advanced bladder cancer: a large, randomized, multicenter trial. ASCO Annual Meeting Proceedings, Chicago, IL. Journal of Clinical Oncology 2003;21(Suppl):391.

[49] Raghavan D, Quinn D, Skinner DG, et al. Surgery and adjunctive chemotherapy for invasive bladder cancer. Surg Oncol 2002;11:55–63.

[50] Collaboration ABCO. Neoadjuvant cisplatin for advanced bladder cancer. Cochrane Database Syst Rev 2000(2):CD001426.

[51] Sternberg CN, Pansadoro V, Calabro F, et al. Can patient selection for bladder preservation be based on response to chemotherapy? Cancer 2003;97: 1644–52.

[52] Collaboration BCM-a. Neoadjuvant chemotherapy in invasive bladder cancer: a systematic review and meta-analysis. Lancet 2003;361:1927–34.

[53] Winquist E, Kirchner TS, Segal R, et al. Neoadjuvant chemotherapy for transitional cell carcinoma of the bladder: a systematic review and meta-analysis. J Urol 2004;171:561–9.

[54] Jordan K, Kasper C, Schmoll HJ. Chemotherapy-induced nausea and vomiting: current and new standards in the antiemetic prophylaxis and treatment. Eur J Cancer 2005;41:199–205.

[55] Grunberg SM. New developments in the management of chemotherapy-induced emesis: do they impact on existing guidelines? Oncology (Huntingt) 2004;18(Suppl 6):15–9.

[56] Smith DB, Newlands ES, Rustin GJ, et al. Comparison of ondansetron and ondansetron plus dexamethasone as antiemetic prophylaxis during cisplatin-containing chemotherapy. Lancet 1991; 338:487–90.

[57] de Wit R, Herrstedt J, Rapoport B, et al. Addition of the oral NK1 antagonist aprepitant to standard antiemetics provides protection against nausea and vomiting during multiple cycles of cisplatin-based chemotherapy. J Clin Oncol 2003;21:4105–11.

[58] Anonymous. American Society of Clinical Oncology. Recommendations for the use of hematopoietic colony-stimulating factors: evidence-based, clinical practice guidelines. J Clin Oncol 1994;12: 2471–508.

[59] Droz J-P, Fizazi K, Beuzeboc P, et al. Gemcitabine and cisplatin (GC) as adjuvant chemotherapy for locally advanced bladder cancer (LABC) after cystectomy: preliminary results of a feasibility study. ASCO Annual Meeting Proceedings, Orlando, Florida. Journal of Clinical Oncology 2002; 20(Suppl):2425.

[60] Meliani E, Lapini A, Serni S, et al. Gemcitabine plus cisplatin in adjuvant regimen for bladder cancer. Toxicity evaluation. Urol Int 2003;71:37–40.

[61] El-Khoueiry AB, Tagawa ST, Vallböhmer D, et al. Adjuvant chemotherapy with gemcitabine and cisplatin for locally advanced transitional cell carcinoma of the bladder (submitted for publication).

[62] Bamias A, Deliveliotis C, Aravantinos G, et al. Adjuvant chemotherapy with paclitaxel and carboplatin in patients with advanced bladder cancer: a study by the Hellenic Cooperative Oncology Group. J Urol 2004;171:1467–70.

[63] Skinner DG, Lieskovsky G. Contemporary cystectomy with pelvic node dissection compared to preoperative radiation therapy plus cystectomy in management of invasive bladder cancer. J Urol 1984;131:1069–72.

[64] Reisinger SA, Mohiuddin M, Mulholland SG. Combined pre- and postoperative adjuvant radiation therapy for bladder cancer—a ten year experience. Int J Radiat Oncol Biol Phys 1992;24: 463–8.

[65] Spera JA, Whittington R, Littman P, et al. A comparison of preoperative radiotherapy regimens for bladder carcinoma. The University of Pennsylvania experience. Cancer 1988;61:255–62.

[66] Ahlering TE, Kanellos A, Boyd SD, et al. A comparative study of perioperative complications with Kock pouch urinary diversion in highly irradiated versus nonirradiated patients. J Urol 1988;139: 1202–4.

[67] Shipley WU, Thames HD, Sandler HM, et al. Radiation therapy for clinically localized prostate cancer: a multi-institutional pooled analysis. JAMA 1999;281:1598–604.

[68] Brown AL Jr, Zietman AL, Shipley WU, et al. An organ-preserving approach to muscle-invading transitional cell cancer of the bladder. Hematol Oncol Clin North Am 2001;15:345–58.

[69] Shipley WU, Kaufman DS, Zehr E, et al. Selective bladder preservation by combined modality protocol treatment: long-term outcomes of 190 patients with invasive bladder cancer. Urology 2002;60: 62–7 [discussion: 67–8].

[70] Kachnic LA, Kaufman DS, Heney NM, et al. Bladder preservation by combined modality therapy for invasive bladder cancer. J Clin Oncol 1997;15: 1022–9.

[71] Eapen L, Stewart D, Collins J, et al. Effective bladder sparing therapy with intra-arterial cisplatin and radiotherapy for localized bladder cancer. J Urol 2004;172:1276–80.

[72] Quek ML, Quinn DI, Daneshmand S, et al. Molecular prognostication in bladder cancer—a current perspective. Eur J Cancer 2003;39:1501–10.

[73] Esrig D, Elmajian D, Groshen S, et al. Accumulation of nuclear p53 and tumor progression in bladder cancer. N Engl J Med 1994;331:1259–64.

[74] Stein JP, Ginsberg DA, Grossfeld GD, et al. Effect of p21WAF1/CIP1 expression on tumor progression in bladder cancer. J Natl Cancer Inst 1998; 90:1072–9.

[75] Cote RJ, Dunn MD, Chatterjee SJ, et al. Elevated and absent pRb expression is associated with bladder cancer progression and has cooperative effects with p53. Cancer Res 1998;58:1090–4.

[76] Chatterjee SJ, Datar R, Youssefzadeh D, et al. Combined effects of p53, p21, and pRb expression in the progression of bladder transitional cell carcinoma. J Clin Oncol 2004;22:1007–13.

[77] Schrag D, Garewal HS, Burstein HJ, et al. American Society of Clinical Oncology Technology Assessment: chemotherapy sensitivity and resistance assays. J Clin Oncol 2004;22:3631–8.

[78] Li L, Elledge SJ, Peterson CA, et al. Specific association between the human DNA repair proteins XPA and ERCC1. Proc Natl Acad Sci U S A 1994;91:5012–6.

[79] Park CH, Bessho T, Matsunaga T, et al. Purification and characterization of the XPF-ERCC1 complex of human DNA repair excision nuclease. J Biol Chem 1995;270:22657–60.

[80] Reed E. Platinum-DNA adduct, nucleotide excision repair and platinum based anti-cancer chemotherapy. Cancer Treat Rev 1998;24:331–44.

[81] Wakasugi M, Sancar A. Assembly, subunit composition, and footprint of human DNA repair excision nuclease. Proc Natl Acad Sci U S A 1998;95: 6669–74.

[82] Sijbers AM, de Laat WL, Ariza RR, et al. Xeroderma pigmentosum group F caused by a defect in a structure-specific DNA repair endonuclease. Cell 1996;86:811–22.

[83] De Silva IU, McHugh PJ, Clingen PH, et al. Defining the roles of nucleotide excision repair and recombination in the repair of DNA interstrand cross-links in mammalian cells. Mol Cell Biol 2000;20:7980–90.

[84] Adair GM, Rolig RL, Moore-Faver D, et al. Role of ERCC1 in removal of long non-homologous tails during targeted homologous recombination. EMBO J 2000;19:5552–61.

[85] Dabholkar M, Bostick-Bruton F, Weber C, et al. ERCC1 and ERCC2 expression in malignant tissues from ovarian cancer patients. J Natl Cancer Inst 1992;84:1512–7.

[86] Dabholkar M, Vionnet J, Bostick-Bruton F, et al. Messenger RNA levels of XPAC and ERCC1 in ovarian cancer tissue correlate with response to platinum-based chemotherapy. J Clin Invest 1994; 94:703–8.

[87] Shirota Y, Stoehlmacher J, Brabender J, et al. ERCC1 and thymidylate synthase mRNA levels predict survival for colorectal cancer patients receiving combination oxaliplatin and fluorouracil chemotherapy. J Clin Oncol 2001;19:4298–304.

[88] Metzger R, Schneider PM, Baldus SE, et al. Quantitative ERCC1 RNA expression identifies nonresponse to cis-platinum based neoadjuvant radiochemotherapy for esophageal cancer. ASCO Annual Meeting Proceedings, San Francisco, CA. Journal of Clinical Oncology 2001;19(Suppl):130.

[89] Metzger R, Leichman CG, Danenberg KD, et al. ERCC1 mRNA levels complement thymidylate synthase mRNA levels in predicting response and survival for gastric cancer patients receiving combination cisplatin and fluorouracil chemotherapy. J Clin Oncol 1998;16:309–16.

[90] Lord RV, Brabender J, Gandara D, et al. Low ERCC1 expression correlates with prolonged survival after cisplatin plus gemcitabine chemotherapy in non-small cell lung cancer. Clin Cancer Res 2002;8:2286–91.

[91] Murray D, Macann A, Hanson J, et al. ERCC1/ ERCC4 5′-endonuclease activity as a determinant of hypoxic cell radiosensitivity. Int J Radiat Biol 1996;69:319–27.

[92] Haffty BG, Glazer PM. Molecular markers in clinical radiation oncology. Oncogene 2003;22: 5915–25.

[93] Tran H, Brunet A, Grenier JM, et al. DNA repair pathway stimulated by the forkhead transcription factor FOXO3a through the Gadd45 protein. Science 2002;296:530–4.

[94] Jiang H, Yang LY. Cell cycle checkpoint abrogator UCN-01 inhibits DNA repair: association with attenuation of the interaction of XPA and ERCC1 nucleotide excision repair proteins. Cancer Res 1999;59:4529–34.

[95] Houtsmuller AB, Rademakers S, Nigg AL, et al. Action of DNA repair endonuclease ERCC1/ XPF in living cells. Science 1999;284:958–61.

[96] Smaletz O, Galsky M, Scher HI, et al. Pilot study of epothilone B analog (BMS-247550) and estramustine phosphate in patients with progressive metastatic prostate cancer following castration. Ann Oncol 2003;14:1518–24.

[97] McDaid HM, Mani S, Shen HJ, et al. Validation of the pharmacodynamics of BMS-247550, an analogue of epothilone B, during a phase I clinical study. Clin Cancer Res 2002;8:2035–43.

[98] Lee Y, Jia Z, Sakowicz R. Inhibitors of the mitotic kinesin KSP: biochemical mechanism of action. Proc Am Soc Cancer Res 2002:A325.

[99] Raymond E, Faivre S, Chaney S, et al. Cellular and molecular pharmacology of oxaliplatin. Mol Cancer Ther 2002;1:227–35.

[100] Stewart CF, Ratain MJ. Topoisomerase interactive agents. In: DeVita VTJ, Hellman S, Rosenberg SA, editors. Cancer: principles and practice of oncol-

ogy. 6th edition. Philadelphia: Lippincott Williams & Wilkins; 2001. p. 415–30.

[101] Kaufmann SH, Peereboom D, Buckwalter CA, et al. Cytotoxic effects of topotecan combined with various anticancer agents in human cancer cell lines. J Natl Cancer Inst 1996;88:734–41.

[102] Tortora G, Caputo R, Damiano V, et al. Combination of a selective cyclooxygenase-2 inhibitor with epidermal growth factor receptor tyrosine kinase inhibitor ZD1839 and protein kinase A antisense causes cooperative antitumor and antiangiogenic effect. Clin Cancer Res 2003;9: 1566–72.

[103] Trifan OC, Durham WF, Salazar VS, et al. Cyclo-oxygenase-2 inhibition with celecoxib enhances antitumor efficacy and reduces diarrhea side effect of CPT-11. Cancer Res 2002;62:5778–84.

[104] Small EJ, Halabi S, Dalbagni G, et al. Overview of bladder cancer trials in the Cancer and Leukemia Group B. Cancer 2003;97(Suppl):2090–8.

[105] Bellmunt J, Hussain M, Dinney CP. Novel approaches with targeted therapies in bladder cancer. Therapy of bladder cancer by blockade of the epidermal growth factor receptor family. Crit Rev Oncol Hematol 2003;46(Suppl):S85–104.

[106] Highshaw RA, McConkey DJ, Dinney CP. Integrating basic science and clinical research in bladder cancer: update from the first bladder Specialized Program of Research Excellence (SPORE). Curr Opin Urol 2004;14:295–300.

[107] Latif Z, Watters AD, Dunn I, et al. HER2/neu gene amplification and protein overexpression in G3 pT2 transitional cell carcinoma of the bladder: a role for anti-HER2 therapy? Eur J Cancer 2004; 40:56–63.

[108] Margolin K, Gordon MS, Holmgren E, et al. Phase Ib trial of intravenous recombinant humanized monoclonal antibody to vascular endothelial growth factor in combination with chemotherapy in patients with advanced cancer: pharmacologic and long-term safety data. J Clin Oncol 2001;19: 851–6.

[109] Levine AM, Quinn DI, Gorospe G, et al. Phase I trial of vascular endothelial growth factor-antisense (VEGF-AS, veglin) in relapsed and refractory malignancies. In: 46th Annual Meeting of the American Society of Hematology, San Diego (CA), December 4–7, 2003. Washington, DC: American Society of Hematology; 2003. p. 418.

[110] Hurwitz H, Fehrenbacher L, Cartwright T, et al. Bevacizumab (a monoclonal antibody to vascular endothelial growth factor) prolongs survival in first-line colorectal cancer (CRC): Results of a phase III trial of bevacizumab in combination with bolus IFL (irinotecan, 5-fluorouracil, leucovorin) as first-line therapy in subjects with metastatic CRC [abstract]. ASCO Annual Meeting Proceedings, Chicago, IL. Journal of Clinical Oncology 2003;21:3646.

[111] Holash J, Davis S, Papadopoulos N, et al. VEGF-Trap: a VEGF blocker with potent antitumor effects. Proc Natl Acad Sci U S A 2002;99: 11393–8.

[112] Abrams TJ, Murray LJ, Pesenti E, et al. Preclinical evaluation of the tyrosine kinase inhibitor SU11248 as a single agent and in combination with "standard of care" therapeutic agents for the treatment of breast cancer. Mol Cancer Ther 2003;2:1011–21.

[113] Schueneman AJ, Himmelfarb E, Geng L, et al. SU11248 maintenance therapy prevents tumor regrowth after fractionated irradiation of murine tumor models. Cancer Res 2003;63:4009–16.

[114] Wood JM, Bold G, Buchdunger E, et al. PTK787/ ZK 222584, a novel and potent inhibitor of vascular endothelial growth factor receptor tyrosine kinases, impairs vascular endothelial growth factor-induced responses and tumor growth after oral administration. Cancer Res 2000;60:2178–89.

[115] Strumberg D, Richly H, Hilger RA, et al. Phase I clinical and pharmacokinetic study of the novel Raf kinase and vascular endothelial growth factor receptor inhibitor BAY 43–9006 in patients with advanced refractory solid tumors. J Clin Oncol 2005;23:965–72.

[116] Wilhelm SM, Carter C, Tang L, et al. BAY 43–9006 exhibits broad spectrum oral antitumor activity and targets the RAF/MEK/ERK pathway and receptor tyrosine kinases involved in tumor progression and angiogenesis. Cancer Res 2004;64:7099–109.

[117] Grossfeld GD, Ginsberg DA, Stein JP, et al. Thrombospondin-1 expression in bladder cancer: association with p53 alterations, tumor angiogenesis, and tumor progression. J Natl Cancer Inst 1997;89:219–27.

[118] Westphal JR. Technology evaluation: ABT-510, Abbott. Curr Opin Mol Ther 2004;6:451–7.

[119] Williams S, Pettaway C, Song R, et al. Differential effects of the proteasome inhibitor bortezomib on apoptosis and angiogenesis in human prostate tumor xenografts. Mol Cancer Ther 2003;2: 835–43.

[120] Ikezoe T, Yang Y, Saito T, et al. Proteasome inhibitor PS-341 down-regulates prostate-specific antigen (PSA) and induces growth arrest and apoptosis of androgen-dependent human prostate cancer LNCaP cells. Cancer Sci 2004;95:271–5.

[121] Cusack JC Jr, Liu R. Enhanced chemosensitivity to CPT-11 with proteasome inhibitor PS-341: implications for systemic nuclear factor-kappaB inhibition. Cancer Res 2001;61:3535–40.

[122] Salem C, Liang G, Tsai YC, et al. Progressive increases in de novo methylation of CpG islands in bladder cancer. Cancer Res 2000;60:2473–6.

[123] Ruefli AA, Ausserlechner MJ, Bernhard D, et al. The histone deacetylase inhibitor and chemotherapeutic agent suberoylanilide hydroxamic acid (SAHA) induces a cell-death pathway characterized

by cleavage of Bid and production of reactive oxygen species. Proc Natl Acad Sci U S A 2001;98: 10833–8.

[124] Richon VM, Zhou X, Rifkind RA, et al. Histone deacetylase inhibitors: development of suberoylanilide hydroxamic acid (SAHA) for the treatment of cancers. Blood Cells Mol Dis 2001;27: 260–4.

[125] Rosato RR, Grant S. Histone deacetylase inhibitors in cancer therapy. Cancer Biol Ther 2003;2:30–7.

[126] Marks P, Rifkind RA, Richon VM, et al. Histone deacetylases and cancer: causes and therapies. Nat Rev Cancer 2001;1:194–202.

[127] Raghavan D. Progress in the chemotherapy of metastatic cancer of the urinary tract. Cancer 2003; 97(Suppl):2050–5.

ELSEVIER
SAUNDERS

Urol Clin N Am 32 (2005) 231–237

UROLOGIC
CLINICS
of North America

Neoadjuvant Chemotherapy in Patients with Invasive Bladder Cancer

David J. Vaughn, MD[a], S. Bruce Malkowicz, MD[b],*

[a]*Division of Hematology/Oncology, Department of Medicine, University of Pennsylvania School of Medicine
and the Abramson Cancer Center of the University of Pennsylvania, 16 Penn Tower,
3400 Spruce Street, Philadelphia, PA 19104, USA*
[b]*Division of Urology, Department of Surgery, University of Pennsylvania School of Medicine
and the Abramson Cancer Center of the University of Pennsylvania, 9 Penn Tower,
3400 Spruce Street, Philadelphia, PA 19104, USA*

This year, approximately 63,210 Americans will be diagnosed with bladder cancer, and an estimated 13,180 Americans will die of this disease [1]. Muscle-invasive bladder cancer is a highly lethal disease with a mortality rate of 70% to 90% over 2 to 3 years if left untreated. Radical cystectomy and bilateral pelvic lymph node dissection can have a significant impact on survival, but outcomes are significantly determined by pathologic stage [2].

In a large series of 1054 patients treated with radical cystectomy and bilateral pelvic lymph node dissection, investigators at the University of Southern California's Norris Comprehensive Cancer Center demonstrated that T and N stage were important predictors of prognosis [3]. These results are shown in Table 1 (the 1987 Tumor-Node-Metastasis (TNM) system was used in this study). For patients who have organ-confined muscle-invasive lymph node–negative disease, the 5- and 10-year survival rates were 89% and 78%, respectively, for pT2 tumors and 87% and 76%, respectively, for pT3a tumors. Patients with extravesical lymph node–negative disease had significantly worse 5- and 10-year survival: 62% and 61%, respectively, for pT3b tumors and 50% and 45%, respectively, for pT4 tumors. The 5- and 10-year survival rates for lymph node–positive disease were 35% and 34%, respectively. While it is clear

from these data that radical cystectomy and pelvic lymph node dissection is an excellent treatment for organ-confined disease, many patients with extravesical or lymph node–positive bladder cancer will develop recurrent disease, often with distant metastases, and will ultimately die of their disease. Given the lethality of muscle-invasive bladder cancer, there is a definite need for effective systemic chemotherapy.

Chemotherapy for advanced urothelial cancer

Bladder cancer is a chemotherapy-sensitive neoplasm. Significant single-agent tumor response rates have been demonstrated with several single agents. Cisplatin-based chemotherapy regimens have been most extensively investigated. In the 1980s, investigators at Memorial Sloan-Kettering Cancer Center (MSKCC) developed the methotrexate, vinblastine, doxorubicin, and cisplatin (MVAC) regimen. Early phase II investigations of MVAC demonstrated tumor response rates in the 70% to 80% range [4]. Subsequently, randomized trials have demonstrated that MVAC is superior to single-agent cisplatin and to CISCA (cyclophosphamide, doxorubicin and cisplatin) [5,6]. The Intergroup evaluated 246 patients with advanced urothelial cancer who were randomized to single agent cisplatin or MVAC. The MVAC arm was associated with a higher tumor response rate and improved overall survival [5]. Investigators at M.D. Anderson Cancer Center randomized patients with advanced bladder cancer to

* Corresponding author.
E-mail address: bruce.malkowicz@uphs.upenn.edu
(S.B. Malkowicz).

Table 1
University of Southern California radical cystectomy series demonstrating optimal effectiveness of surgery in the treatment of muscle-invasive disease

Pathology (using 1987 Tumor-Node-Metastasis system)	Survival	
	5-year (%)	10-year (%)
pT0	92	86
PTis	91	89
PTa	79	74
pT1	83	78
pT2N0	89	78
pT3aN0	87	76
pT3bN0	62	61
pT4N0	50	45
N + 1–4	35	34
N + ≥5	31	23

MVAC versus CISCA and, again, MVAC was associated with an improved tumor response rate and survival [6]. Based on these randomized trials, MVAC emerged as the standard chemotherapy regimen for patients who have metastatic bladder cancer.

However, MVAC is associated with significant toxicity including mucositis, myelosuppression, and renal dysfunction [4–6]. Some of these toxicities can be abrogated with the prophylactic use of granulocyte–colony-stimulating factor (G-CSF) [7]. More recently, high-dose intensity MVAC has been compared with standard MVAC in a recently reported trial by the European Organization for the Research and Treatment of Cancer (EORTC) [8]. High-dose intensity MVAC employs the same doses of the MVAC drugs, but are cycled more frequently using G-CSF. Compared with MVAC, the high-dose intensity MVAC regimen resulted in improved tolerability and similar survival.

Recently, novel agents such as gemcitabine and the taxanes have been studied extensively in bladder cancer. A Phase III trial compared a combination of gemcitabine and cisplatin to MVAC in patients with advanced urothelial cancer [9]. This international industry-sponsored trial accrued 405 patients, the largest bladder cancer chemotherapy trial to date. This trial demonstrated that the overall survival of patients treated with gemcitabine/cisplatin was similar to those treated with MVAC (the trial was not sufficiently powered to prove equivalency of the 2 regimens). However, MVAC was associated with significantly greater risk of grade 3 to 4 mucositis, granulocytopenia, fever, and sepsis. Gemcitabine/cisplatin was associated with significantly more grade 3 to 4 anemia and thrombocytopenia. It should be noted that the MVAC group did not receive prophylactic G-CSF in this trial. The results of this trial established gemcitabine/cisplatin as an alternative to MVAC for patients who have advanced bladder cancer.

How effective is cisplatin-based combination chemotherapy in patients with metastatic urothelial cancer with respect to long-term survival? Which patients are most likely to derive long-term benefit? Bajorin and colleagues [10] analyzed a group of 203 patients with advanced bladder cancer treated with MVAC to determine risk factors that predict survival. The presence of visceral (defined as lung, liver, or bone) metastases and a baseline Karnofsky performance status of less than 80% predicted independently for a poor outcome. Patients that had both of these risk factors had a 5-year survival of 0% (median survival 9.3 months). However, if patients had neither risk factor, the chance of 5-year survival was 33% (median survival 33 months). At 6-year follow-up of the previously described Intergroup trial of MVAC versus cisplatin [5], only 3.7% of patients treated with MVAC experienced long-term cancer-free survival. Predictors for worsened survival in this study included nontransitional histology, poor performance status, or bone or visceral metastasis [11]. Thus it is clear that while the chance for long-term survival for most patients with metastatic urothelial cancer treated with MVAC is small, the most favorable prognosis patients are those with preserved performance status and nodal/nonvisceral metastases.

Neoadjuvant versus adjuvant chemotherapy

To increase surgical cure rates for highly lethal diseases such as muscle-invasive bladder cancer, systemic chemotherapy may be administered to patients either before (neoadjuvant) or after (adjuvant) definitive local treatments. If one considers that cisplatin-based combination chemotherapy in metastatic bladder cancer is most efficacious in patients with preserved performance status and nodal/nonvisceral disease [10,11], then employing these drugs in the minimal disease neoadjuvant or adjuvant setting seems rationale.

The advantages of neoadjuvant chemotherapy include the potential for primary tumor downstaging, the early systemic exposure of cytotoxic agents, and the potential for decreased toxicity in the patient before surgery. In addition, neoadjuvant chemotherapy affords the opportunity to determine chemosensitivity of the tumor, which may have prognostic significance and direct further therapies. The advantages of adjuvant therapy include the ability to select patients for treatment based on definitive pathological stage so as not to "overtreat" patients. In addition, adjuvant therapy does not result in the delay of definitive surgical treatment, which some consider a disadvantage of the neoadjuvant approach.

Downstaging bladder cancer with neoadjuvant chemotherapy

Because bladder cancer is chemosensitive, neoadjuvant chemotherapy may result in a significant response of the primary tumor. In some cases, tumor downstaging with neoadjuvant chemotherapy can result in patients who had previously unresectable disease (eg, tumors fixed to the pelvic sidewall) ultimately undergoing cystectomy [12]. The degree of tumor response to neoadjuvant chemotherapy also carries prognostic importance. In a trial from MSKCC, 125 patients with muscle-invasive disease were treated with cisplatin-based chemotherapy followed by surgery. For responding patients (defined as $\leq$pT1 at cystectomy), 91% were disease-free compared with only 37% of nonresponders ($\geq$pT2 at cystectomy) [13]. Prognostic factors for survival for patients treated with neoadjuvant chemotherapy include initial tumor stage and postchemotherapy pathologic stage, consistent with the extent of chemotherapy downstaging [13,14].

Select patients with an excellent response of the primary tumor to neoadjuvant chemotherapy may be candidates for a more conservative surgical approach such as repeat transurethral resections or partial cystectomy [12]. In an MSKCC series of 111 patients treated with neoadjuvant MVAC, 26 underwent partial cystectomy [15]. At a median follow-up of 6.9 years, 17 (65%) of the 26 patients were alive. Fourteen (54%) patients had a functioning bladder. It must be remembered that patients who have their bladders preserved using this approach have an approximately 50% chance of developing new bladder cancers up to 10 years later [16].

In addition, molecular biomarkers may potentially identify patients who are more likely to fare well with a neoadjuvant bladder-preserving approach. In an MSKCC study of 90 patients treated with neoadjuvant chemotherapy, p53 status of the tumors predicted survival [17]. Patients who had wild-type p53 (negative nuclear staining by way of immunohistochemical analysis) had significantly better survival rates than patients who had mutant p53 (>20% nuclear staining). Patients with T2 and T3a tumors that expressed wild-type p53 did especially well, with a 5-year survival rate of 77%. Based on this data, a follow-up MSKCC trial is currently examining the role of bladder preservation in these favorable prognosis tumors. Patients with nonobstructing T2/T3a tumors that are wild-type for p53 are treated with transurethral resection of the tumor followed by neoadjuvant MVAC. Patients in a complete response are observed; patients with an incomplete response undergo salvage cystectomy [18]. This trial complements an onging prospective international trial in which patients with organ-confined disease on final pathology are evaluated for p53 status and then randomized to adjuvant chemotherapy. This effort will shed further insight regarding the association of p53 expression and chemotherapy response as well as the ability to identify high-risk populations among patients with organ-confined disease by means of a biomarker.

Does neoadjuvant chemotherapy improve survival in invasive bladder cancer?

As discussed, neoadjuvant chemotherapy can play an important role in downstaging bladder tumors. However, does neoadjuvant chemotherapy improve survival in patients with muscle-invasive disease? This question has been extensively studied.

Meta-analyses examining the randomized controlled trials of neoadjuvant chemotherapy bladder cancer have been performed. The most recent systematic review and meta-analysis has been reported by Winquist and colleagues [19] and the Genitourinary Cancer Disease Site Group of Cancer Care Ontario Program in Evidence-Based Care Practice Guidelines Initiative. This group performed a systematic review and meta-analysis of all known randomized controlled trials of neoadjuvant chemotherapy for muscle-invasive bladder cancer. The group identified 16 randomized controlled trials of neoadjuvant chemotherapy for invasive bladder cancer that included a total of 3315 eligible randomized patients. In addition, data from previously published meta-analyses were used. Given inconsistencies and incomplete data from some trials, a total of 11 trials with a total of 2605 patients were ultimately examined. The pooled hazard ratio from these 11 trials was 0.90 (95% CI 0.82–0.99; $P = .02$). This result was consistent with a 10% decrease in the risk of death or an absolute survival advantage of 5.0% (95% CI 0.0.5–9.0) from 50% to 55%. When the 8 trials that used cisplatin-based combination chemotherapy were examined, the pooled hazard ratio was 0.87 (95% CI 0.78–0.96; $P = .006$). This hazard ratio was consistent with an absolute survival advantage of 6.5% (95% CI 2%–11%) from 50 to 56.5%. Interestingly, when the 3 trials that used single-agent cisplatin were examined (a total of 337 patients), the survival benefit was not demonstrated. The meta-analysis of the randomized controlled trials of neoadjuvant chemotherapy in bladder cancer did not show statistical heterogeneity, and the authors report that the hazard ratios are of a "fixed effect model." Overall, the rate of chemotherapy-related mortality was 1.1%. Therefore, this meta-analysis demonstrates that cisplatin-based chemotherapy improves survival in muscle-invasive bladder cancer.

Lessons from one trial: INT-0080

The United States Intergroup (INT)-0080 trial [20] was reported in 2003. In INT-0080, 317 patients with T2-T4a bladder cancer were randomized to 3 cycles of neoadjuvant MVAC followed by cystectomy versus cystectomy alone. Using intention-to-treat analysis, the median survival of patients in the cystectomy alone arm was 46 months versus 77 months in the neoadjuvant chemotherapy plus cystectomy arm ($P = .06$ by two-sided stratified log-rank test). There are several issues of interest that are demonstrated in the trial. First, complete downstaging to a no residual disease status at cystectomy had a significant impact on survival. More patients in the neoadjuvant chemotherapy plus cystectomy group demonstrated no residual cancer (that is, pT0 disease status) than in the cystectomy alone arm (38% vs 15%; $P < .001$). The survival benefit of a pT0 disease status in patients treated with neoadjuvant chemotherapy

or cystectomy alone was significant, with 85% and 82% of patients alive at 5 years, respectively. Second, patients enrolled in the trial were stratified by initial tumor stage (T2 vs T3 or T4a) and age (<65 years vs ≥ 65 years). Neither initial stage nor patient age had a significant effect on survival. Finally, the administration of neoadjuvant MVAC did not prevent patients from undergoing radical cystectomy, nor was it associated with more surgery-related complications. In fact, unlike trials of the MVAC combination in metastatic bladder cancer, there were no chemotherapy-related deaths. It is not clear whether this was related to increased familiarity of the regimen by the treating oncologists, better performance status and health of the patients being treated, or simply chance.

The importance of surgical factors in examining the results of neoadjuvant chemotherapy in bladder cancer

An important supplemental analysis of the INT-0080 trial demonstrated the importance of considering surgical factors when evaluating large cystectomy chemotherapy trials [21]. Patients who had complete surgical records and who underwent cystectomy according to protocol were analyzed (n = 268). The cystectomies were performed by 106 surgeons at 109 institutions. Half of the patients received neoadjuvant chemotherapy.

Five-year postcystectomy survival rates were 54%, and local recurrence rates were 15%. In a multivariate model adjusted for MVAC administration, age, pathologic stage, and node status demonstrated that surgical variables associated with longer postcystectomy survival included negative surgical margins (Hazard Ratio (HR) 0.37; $P = .0007$) and 10 or more nodes removed (HR 0.51; $P = .0001$). These associations did not vary by treatment arms ($P > .21$). Predictors of local recurrence in adjusted multivariate models were positive margins (odds ratio 11.2; $P = .0001$) and fewer than 10 nodes removed (odds ratio 5.1; $P = .002$). The conclusion of this analysis was that surgical factors can influence cystectomy outcomes apart from pathologic factors or neoadjuvant treatment status. Thus the extent and uniformity of cystectomy and bilateral pelvic lymph node dissection is a factor to be considered in trials involving the perioperative use of chemotherapy.

Neoadjuvant chemotherapy for bladder cancer in perspective

Selected randomized controlled cisplatin-based combination chemotherapy trials demonstrate survival benefit, which is supported by a recently published meta-analysis [19]. These data on neoadjuvant chemotherapy do not irrefutably establish this sequence of therapy as the new standard of care for patients with muscle-invasive bladder cancer. Randomized trials of adjuvant chemotherapy in bladder cancer have also been performed [22]. Although these trials suffer in general from being underpowered and problematic with respect to trial methodology, two trials suggest survival benefit [23,24]. Presently, the EORTC and the SWOG are conducting a randomized trial of adjuvant chemotherapy in high-risk bladder cancer patients. This trial randomizes patients with pT3 or pT4 or node-positive bladder cancer to either early postoperative chemotherapy versus chemotherapy deferred until the time of disease progression. The chemotherapy regimens that are being evaluated include MVAC, high-dose intensity MVAC, and gemcitabine/cisplatin. With an overall accrual goal of 1344 patients, the trial is sufficiently powered to demonstrate a 5% survival difference at 5 years.

Is there an advantage to preoperative neoadjuvant chemotherapy as opposed to postoperative adjuvant chemotherapy in bladder cancer? In an important study examining this issue in bladder cancer, Millikan and colleagues [25] randomized 140 patients with muscle-invasive disease to two cycles of neoadjuvant MVAC chemotherapy followed by cystectomy plus pelvic lymph node dissection, followed by three more cycles of adjuvant MVAC; or to cystectomy followed by five cycles of adjuvant MVAC chemotherapy. Of note, at a median follow-up of almost 6 years, 58% of all patients were alive and disease-free. However, there was no statistically significant difference in survival between the two arms. This is consistent with trials in other chemotherapy-sensitive disease sites (eg, the breast) that have not proven a survival advantage to neoadjuvant chemotherapy over adjuvant treatment [26].

It is with caution that we must point out that most of the newer non–cisplatin-based chemotherapy regimens, and even the gemcitabine/cisplatin regimen, which are currently being used in metastatic disease, have not been evaluated in the adjuvant or neoadjuvant setting. It should not be assumed that all regimens are the same as MVAC. However, the ongoing EORTC/SWOG adjuvant trial incorporates MVAC, high-dose intensity MVAC, and gemcitabine/cisplatin in the adjuvant chemotherapy arm.

Currently the literature concerning perioperative chemotherapy—be it neoadjuvant or adjuvant—when viewed as a whole provides strong support for the use of perioperative chemotherapy in patients with poor-risk bladder cancer who are to undergo cystectomy. At the Abramson Cancer Center of the University of Pennsylvania, our general approach is to discuss the available information on perioperative therapy with cystectomy candidates. Those with bulky, local disease are encouraged to consider neoadjuvant therapy, while individuals with low-volume/stage disease usually undergo cystectomy. The use of adjuvant therapy is based on pathological findings and the patient's overall general health status. If a patient has pT3 or pT4 or node-positive disease, and can tolerate chemotherapy, we will offer the patient four cycles of adjuvant cisplatin-based chemotherapy (either MVAC or the gemcitabine/cisplatin, two regimens with similar efficacy in the advanced disease setting). However, we make clear in our discussion with the patient that our recommendation is based on supportive but not definitive evidence, and that it is the best we can offer until more definitive data are available (eg, the ongoing EORTC/SWOG trial).

Summary

Neoadjuvant chemotherapy has been extensively investigated in muscle-invasive bladder cancer. When taken together, the randomized controlled trials of neoadjuvant cisplatin-based combination chemotherapy demonstrate an improved survival over cystectomy alone. In addition, neoadjuvant chemotherapy can result in downstaging of primary tumors. As noted, a pT0 disease status at cystectomy is associated with a significant improvement in survival. A randomized controlled trial comparing neoadjuavnt to adjuvant cisplatin-based chemotherapy shows that neither approach is superior. Finally, the ongoing EORTC/SWOG adjuvant chemotherapy trial, when completed, should add importantly to the literature concerning the role of systemic chemotherapy in muscle-invasive bladder cancer.

References

[1] Jemal A, Taylor M, Ward E, et al. Cancer statistics, 2005. CA Cancer J Clin 2005;55:10–30.

[2] Frazier HA, Robertson E, Dodge RK, et al. The value of pathologic factors in predicting cancer specific survival among patients treated with radical cystectomy for transitional cell carcinoma of the bladder and the prostate. Cancer 1993;71: 3993–4001.

[3] Stein JP, Lieskovsky G, Richard C, et al. Radical cystectomy in the treatment of invasive bladder cancer: long-term results in 1,054 patients. J Clin Oncol 2001;19:666–75.

[4] Sternberg CN, Yagoda A, Scher HI, et al. Methotrexate, vinblastine, doxorubicin, and cisplatin for advanced transitional cell carcinoma of the urothelium: efficacy and patterns of response and relapse. Cancer 1989;64:2448–58.

[5] Loehrer PJ Sr, Einhorn LH, Elson PJ, et al. A randomized comparison of cisplatin alone or in combination with methotrexate, vinblastine, and doxorubicin in patients with metastatic urothelial carcinoma: a Cooperative Group study. J Clin Oncol 1992;10:1066–73.

[6] Logothetis CJ, Dries FH, Sell A, et al. A prospective randomized trial comparing CISCA to MVAC chemotherapy in advanced metastatic urothelial tumors. J Clin Oncol 1990;8:1050–5.

[7] Gabrilove JL, Jakubowski A, Scher H, et al. Effect of granulocyte colony-stimulating factor on neutropenia and associated morbidity due to chemotherapy for transitional cell carcinoma of the urothelium. N Engl J Med 1988;318:1414–22.

[8] Sternberg CN, de Mulder PHM, Schomagel JH, et al. Randomized phase III trial of high-dose-intensity methotrexate, vinblastine, doxorubicin, and cisplatin (MVAC) chemotherapy and recombinant human granulocyte colony-stimulating factor versus classic MVAC in advanced urothelial tract tumors: European Organization for Research and Treatment Protocol No. 30924. J Clin Oncol 2001;19: 2638–46.

[9] von der Maase H, Hansen SW, Roberts JT, et al. Gemcitabine and cisplatin versus methotrexate, vinblastine, doxorubicin, and cisplatin in advanced or metastatic bladder cancer: results of a large, randomized, multinational, multicenter, phase III study. J Clin Oncol 2000;18:3068–77.

[10] Bajorin DF, Dodd PM, Mazumdar M, et al. Long-term survival in metastatic transitional cell carcinoma and prognostic factors predicting outcome to chemotherapy. J Clin Oncol 1999;17: 3173–81.

[11] Saxman SB, Propert KJ, Einhorn LH, et al. Long-term follow-up of a phase III intergroup study of cisplatin alone or in combination with methotrexate, vinblastine, and doxorubicin in patients with metastatic urothelial carcinoma: a cooperative group study. J Clin Oncol 1997;15:2564–9.

[12] Sternberg CN, Pansadoro V. Chemotherapy and conservative surgery. In: Vogelzang NJ, Scardino PT, Shipley WU, et al, editors. Comprehensive textbook of genitourinary oncology. 2nd edition. Philadelphia: Lippincott Williams & Wilkins; 2000. p. 496–505.

[13] Splinter TA, Scher HI, Denis L, et al. The prognostic value of pathological response to combination chemotherapy before cystectomy in patients with invasive bladder cancer. J Urol 1992;147: 606–8.

[14] Scher H, Herr H, Sternberg C, et al. Neoadjuvant chemotherapy for invasive bladder cancer: experience with the M-VAC regimen. Br J Urol 1989;64: 250–6.

[15] Herr HW, Scher HI. Neoadjuvant chemotherapy and partial cystectomy for invasive bladder cancer. J Clin Oncol 1994;12:975–80.

[16] Herr HW, Bajorin DF, Scher HI. Neoadjuvant chemotherapy and bladder-sparing surgery for invasive bladder cancer: ten-year outcome. J Clin Oncol 1998;16:1298–301.

[17] Sarkis AB, Bajorin DF, Reuter VE, et al. Prognostic value of p53 nuclear overexpression in patients with invasive bladder cancer treated with neoadjuvant MVAC. J Clin Oncol 1995;13: 1384–90.

[18] McCaffrey JA, Bajorin DF. Adjuvant and neoadjuvant chemotherapy for invasive urothelial carcinoma. In: Vogelzang NJ, Scardino PT, Shipley WU, et al, editors. Comprehensive textbook of genitourinary oncology. 2nd edition. Philadelphia: Lippincott Williams & Wilkins; 2000. p. 473–82.

[19] Winquist E, Kirchner TS, Segal R, et al. Genitourinary cancer disease site group, cancer care Ontario program in evidence-based care practice guidelines initiative. J Urol 2004;171:561–9.

[20] Grossman H, Natale R, Tangen C, et al. Neoadjuvant chemotherapy plus cystectomy compared with cystectomy alone for locally advanced bladder cancer. N Engl J Med 2003;349:859–66.

[21] Herr HW, Faulkner JR, Grossman HB, et al. Surgical factors influence bladder cancer outcomes: a cooperative group trial. J Clin Oncol 2004;22: 2781–9.

[22] Dimopoulos MA, Moulopoulos LA. Role of adjuvant chemotherapy in the treatment of invasive carcinoma of the urinary bladder. J Clin Oncol 1998;16:1601–12.

[23] Skinner DG, Daniels, Russell CA, et al. The role of adjuvant chemotherapy following cystectomy for invasive bladder cancer: a prospective comparative trial. J Urol 1991;145:459–67.

[24] Stockle M, Meyenburg W, Wellek S, et al. Advanced bladder cancer: improved survival after radical cystectomy and 3 adjuvant cycles of chemotherapy.

Results of a controlled prospective study. J Urol 1992;148:302–7.

[25] Millikan R, Dinney C, Swanson D, et al. Integrated therapy for locally advanced bladder cancer: final report of a randomized trial of cystectomy plus adjuvant M-VAC versus cystectomy with both pre-operative and postoperative M-VAC. J Clin Oncol 2001;19:4005–13.

[26] Fisher B, Bryant J, Wolmark N, et al. Effect of pre-operative chemotherapy on the outcome of women with operable breast cancer. J Clin Oncol 1998;16: 2672–85.

ELSEVIER
SAUNDERS

Urol Clin N Am 32 (2005) 239–246

UROLOGIC
CLINICS
of North America

Clinical Applications for Targeted Therapy in Bladder Cancer

Liana Adam, MD, PhD, Wassim Kassouf, MD, Colin P.N. Dinney, MD*

The University of Texas M.D. Anderson Cancer Center, Departments of Urology and Cancer Biology, 1515 Holcombe Boulevard, Unit 1373, Houston, TX 77030, USA

Transitional cell carcinoma (TCC) of the bladder is the fourth most common solid-tumor malignancy in men in the United States. Approximately 17,060 men in the United States died from TCC of the bladder in 2004; most of the deaths were due to metastatic disease [1]. Metastatic TCC is usually treated with systemic chemotherapy, including regimens such as M-VAC (methotrexate, vinblastine, doxorubicin, and cisplatin) [2–4]. However, despite systemic chemotherapy with even the most effective regimens, most patients with distant metastatic bladder cancer die of the disease after a median survival duration of 18 months [3,4]. Although considerable efforts have been made to escalate the dose of M-VAC, to modulate the components of the regimens, and to use novel combination regimens that include active agents such as paclitaxel, gemcitabine, and ifosfamide, there has been no improvement in survival [5–10]. Although some of these newer regimens produce fewer toxic side effects than M-VAC, there is yet no compelling evidence that they improve patient survival.

In general, the treatment of metastatic TCC of the bladder by classic cytotoxic chemotherapy has reached a therapeutic plateau. Despite high rates of response to treatment, the disease is generally incurable. However, it is clear that cytotoxic chemotherapy has provided significant palliation for many patients, and has resulted in improved outcome, probability for cure, or both in the adjuvant setting of microscopic metastatic disease.

Although chemotherapy is still an important component of combined therapy, the need for more effective treatment options exists. Fortunately, an improved understanding of the biology of malignancy is finally facilitating the design of novel therapeutic approaches to battle cancer.

Urothelial transformation involves several cellular events including the deregulation of cell-cycle and apoptotic pathways via mutation or altered expression of p53, p21/WAF-1, pRB, p27, and INK4A (p16). Progression of urothelial carcinoma has also been related to various members of the erbB family, vascular epidermal growth factor (VEGF), nerve factor-kappa B (NFκB), Akt, PTEN, and cyclooxygenase/2 (COX-2) [11]. All of these molecules are potential targets for novel therapies. The focus of this article is the aberrant signal transduction of members of the erbB family (ie, epidermal growth factor receptor [EGFR], and human epidermal growth factor receptors [HER]-2, -3, and -4) in TCC of the bladder.

EGFR was sequenced and cloned by Ullrich in 1984 [12]. EGFR, HER1, or c-erbB1, is the prototype of the type I receptor tyrosine kinase (RTK) family, which also includes HER2 (c-erbB2), HER3 (c-erbB-3), and HER4 (c-erbB-4) [13–15]. EGFR family members transmit the biologic effects of the EGF family of ligands, which includes EGF, transforming growth factor-α (TGFα), amphiregulin, heparin-binding (HB)-EGF, betacellulin, and epiregulin. Ligand binding induces the formation of homodimers or heterodimers between EGFR and other members of this family, autophosphorylation of tyrosine residues in its intracellular domain, and activation of downstream signaling pathways [13–15]. These

---

* Corresponding author.
E-mail address: cdinney@mdanderson.org
(C.P.N. Dinney).

phosphotyrosines, in turn, phosphorylate other intracellular proteins that contain src homologous domains (SH2 and SH3), such as ras-associated GTPase activating protein, phosphatidylinositol-3-kinase, and phospholipase Cγ. The downstream signaling pathways activated by these intracellular proteins include the ras/raf MAPKinase, phosphatidylinositol-3-kinase, and protein kinase C pathways, which ultimately lead to increased nuclear transcription and subsequent cellular proliferation [15,16].

Overexpression of EGFR alone or accompanied by production of one or more of its ligands, such as TGFα, has been reported in a range of human malignancies and is often associated with poor prognosis [16,17]. Overexpression of EGFR in bladder cancer has been widely reported [18–23]. The reports suggest the presence of erbB1 in 23% to 100% of TCC samples. Several studies have shown that EGFR is positively associated with advanced tumor stage, tumor progression, and poor clinical outcome [24]. Immunohistochemical analyses suggest that rather than actual overexpression of erbB1 in TCC is the actual change in the distribution of the molecule, from basal layer in normal urothelium to all layers in premalignant or malignant urotheliums [25,26]. Other studies have demonstrated that expression of erbB1 and of erbB2 is downregulated in TCC compared with the expression in normal urothelium [27]. Still other studies have demonstrated erbB3 in 20% to 56% and erbB4 in 11% to 30% of cases of TCC, but reduced expression of erbB3 and erbB4 in TCC compared with normal tissues [27]. Statistical analyses of erbB expression patterns and clinical parameters have resulted in varying conclusions about the prognostic significance of erbB expression in TCC [27–32]. However, in patients with muscle-invasive TCC of the bladder, a retrospective immunohistochemical study has shown erbB2 overexpression to be an independent predictor of reduced cancer-specific survival [33]. In contrast, another prospective study found that erbB2 overexpression in the context of paclitaxel-based chemotherapy significantly decreased the risk of death [34].

On the basis of discovery of variant isoforms of the erbB family members, a series of studies was initiated that focused on acquiring quantitative information about erbB status, which was considered critical for selecting patients for erbB inhibitor therapies, and for evaluating the potential use of erbBs as prognostic indicators for patients with cancer. A report by Juntilla et al [35] describing specific erbB4 cytoplasmic or juxtamembrane isoforms overexpressed in TCC compared with its expression in interstitial cystitis or normal bladder, is an example of such finding. Thus, preclinical evidence about the expression levels of specific erbBs in TCC tissues, although controversial at the moment, may be verified through a more refined investigation. Several erbB1 variants, somatic mutations, deletions, or truncations have been described for erbB1 in epithelial cancers, including lung, colon, and breast cancers [36–39]. For example, the erbBvIII variant, which lacks the extracellular domain, has been shown to be specifically expressed in tumor tissues rather than in normal, adjacent tissues and to activate aberrant signaling pathways relevant for EGFR-targeted therapy [40,41]. However, there currently are no studies investigating this aspect in bladder cancer.

Unconventional mechanisms of erbBs signals

Although many of the changes elicited by erbB1 signaling cascades occur in the cytosol, growth factor receptor signaling greatly affects nuclear events such as mitogenesis and changes in transcription. Until recently, these signals were thought to be transmitted through multistep cascades. Eight years ago, a new mode of growth factor receptor signaling to the nucleus was discerned when it was reported that EGFR directly activates the signal transducers and activators of transcription (STAT) proteins [42] or may act as a transcription regulator through direct chromatin binding [43]. Despite nearly a decade of further evidence supporting these data, the mechanistic basis of these perplexing findings has never been discovered. Important questions regarding how the molecule arrived at the nucleus and how it functioned needed to be answered to facilitate the acceptance by the scientific community.

During the past 4 years, new work has been generated to support a simple explanation for the first question: Secreted growth factors gain entry to the nucleus by binding to their cognate receptors. This suggestion introduces a new question: How do receptors move from the plasma membrane to the nucleus, an event that requires not only translocation to another compartment but also liberation from a lipid bilayer? Acidic and basic fibroblastic growth factor (FGF) ligands might constitute a special case, because they lack the classic signal sequences that direct secretion. These growth factors are present in the cytosol, and may move to the nucleus through routine nuclear-import channels without having to gain entry to the cell using their receptors. Changes in receptor hydrophobicity have been described in nuclear translocated insulin growth factor receptor or erbB2 in certain circumstances [44,45]. Complex formation between erbB4 and STAT5A with chaperone-like activity masking the hydrophobicity of the membrane-spanning region to allow membrane escape, transport, or both to the nucleus has recently been described in a breast model [46].

Another intriguing possibility for the role of ligands comes from the recent discovery of matricrine signaling, that is, signaling by extracellular matrix protein domains through direct binding to classic growth factor receptors [47]. The study showed that ultralow affinity and seemingly cryptic ligands for EGFRs are encoded within integral matrix components (tenascin-C through its EGF-like domains). These ligands might be limited in receptor responses such that they cannot induce nuclear translocation and subsequent cellular responses. Alternatively, it has also been proposed that if such matrikines promote nuclear translocation, their role might be simply to initiate the process at the plasma membrane.

One such example, which involves human TCC of the bladder in particular, is HB-EGF, a multifunctional member of the EGF family. HB-EGF is initially synthesized as a membrane-anchored precursor, proHB-EGF, which can participate in juxtacrine interactions with EGFR, the erbB4 RTK expressed on adjacent cells or both leading to receptor activation and increased cell–cell adhesion. On the other hand, soluble HB-EGF mediates paracrine and autocrine activation of the same receptors. A recent study demonstrated that proHB-EGF could be localized to the nucleus, in which case it represents an important feature of aggressive TCC [48].

Constitutive receptor activation caused by overexpression or autocrine growth factor stimulation as well as aberrant downstream signaling has been linked to the development of hyperproliferative diseases such as cancer [49]. In addition, EGFR has been shown to be activated by heterologous extracellular stimuli such as cell adhesion molecules, cytokine receptors, stress agents, and G-protein–coupled receptors (GPCRs) [50]. Recently, several groups have demonstrated the involvement of EGF-like precursor cleavage by metalloproteinase activity in EGFR transactivation pathways [51–55]. These

new mechanisms combined with the classic mechanisms of EGFR signaling emphasize the importance of EGFR as a tumor cell's "mastermind molecule."

The multiple biologic consequences of EGFR activation include increased cell proliferation, reduced apoptosis, increased angiogenesis, increased motility, tumor invasion, and metastasis. Receptor blockade by antibodies or small molecular-weight RTK inhibitors has been shown to inhibit tumor-cell proliferation, induce terminal differentiation, promote apoptosis, and inhibit angiogenesis and metastasis of EGFR-overexpressed tumors both in vitro and in vivo. Among the armamentarium of drugs that target members of the erbB family are, trastuzumab (Herceptin; Genentech, San Francisco, California) and gefitinib (Iressa; Astra Zeneca, United Kingdom) for which phase III trails have been completed.

In one trial, trastuzumab plus chemotherapy was demonstrated to produce longer time to disease progression than chemotherapy alone in women with metastatic breast cancer and of erbB2 overexpression [56]. Furthermore, trastuzumab alone has been associated with a 15% response rate in patients with metastatic erbB-positive breast cancer [57]. Precise identification of erbB2 status is important because patients who would benefit most from trastuzumab-based therapy can be accurately selected, obviating the risk of trastuzumab-induced myocardial dysfunction syndrome in those who would not benefit from the drug.

Another biologic therapy agent, gefitinib, has been demonstrated to be clinically safe when combined with cisplatin/gemcitabine and carboplatin/paclitaxel in the treatment of lung cancer [58]. These combination regimens have been conducted in two multicenter, multinational phase III trials as first-line treatment for patients with inoperable stage III/IV non–small-cell lung cancer. Patients received gefitinib (250 mg or 500 mg daily) in combination with standard regimens of cisplatin, gemcitabine (the INTACT 1 trial) or carboplatin/paclitaxel (INTACT 2 trial). Unexpectedly, these trials did not confirm the synergy of these drug combinations in preclinical models [59–61]. Interestingly, in a recent study, tumors that were sensitive to gefitinib had an EGFR mutation, which may explain why the majority of the tumors in the study did not respond to the EGFR blocker [36,37]. Screening for this mutation in bladder cancer might identify patients who are appropriate candidates for gefitinib therapy.

A review of the results of 200 studies involving more than 20,000 patients revealed a strong (over 70%) prognostic value for head and neck, ovarian, cervical, bladder, and esophageal cancers but a weak (30%) prognostic value in non–small-cell lung cancer. Nonetheless, we now know that some patients with high levels of EGFR expression are refractory to EGFR inhibitor treatment, suggesting that expression of EGFR alone is not a robust predictor of response to therapy. Preclinical studies on 60 cell lines of the United States National Cancer Institute Anticancer Drug Screen were performed with a panel of 11 selective erbB inhibitors. Cell lines expressing high levels of EGFR were divided into two groups: those that were sensitive or insensitive to EGFR inhibitors, and those that were not [62]. This study showed that the level of EGFR expression for the specific tumor was less important than the degree of EGFR activation in predicting response to targeted therapy. Factors affecting activation status included receptor mutation, heterodimerization, and increased expression of ligands [62]. Thus, signaling complexity caused by the interactions among four receptors and 10 ligands makes it difficult to definitively measure signaling output for individual human tumors [63]. When this finding is considered in combination with EGFR transactivation through insulin growth factor receptor (IGFR), platelet-derived growth factor receptor (PDGFR), GPCR, matrikine signaling, or nuclear translocation, it is obvious how complicated it is to make a simple prediction about the clinical effectiveness of targeted therapies.

Inhibition of epidermal growth factor receptor in bladder cancer

Several monoclonal antibodies (mAbs) directed against EGFR are in various stages of clinical development [63] and have the following mechanisms of action: extracellular binding, internalization of the inactive receptor, inhibition of EGFR-generated downstream signals, and potential stimulation of an immunologic response. The most extensively studied of the anti-EGFR mAbs in bladder cancer is cetuximab (Erbitux or C225, a chimeric mAb designed to specifically inhibit EGFR) [64,65]. Using the highly tumorigenic, EGFR-overexpressing 253J B-V cells [65] was shown to downregulate VEGF, interleukin-8 (IL-8), and bFGF expression in tumor xenografts and the involution of tumor blood vessels was

shown to be responsible for an often more pronounced effect in xenograft models than in cell culture. However, this in vivo effect was not observed in cells that were resistant in vitro as well, suggesting that other mechanisms of resistance may actually be responsible for this phenomenon (Dinney, unpublished observations).

The tyrosine-kinase-inhibitors (TKIs) are synthetic, mainly quinazoline-derived small molecules that interact with the intracellular tyrosine kinase domain of several receptors, including EGFR, and inhibit receptor phosphorylation by competing for the intracellular Mg-ATP-binding site [63]. Gefitinib inhibits the kinase activity of isolated EGFR with an IC_{50} in the nanomolar range [56,63], although it seems that, due to the high intracellular concentration of ATP, higher concentrations may be required to inhibit kinase activity in vivo. At micromolar concentrations, gefitinib inhibits other tyrosine kinase receptors, including erbB2 [63].

In studies on cell lines and xenografts other than the bladder, no simple correlation between EGFR expression and sensitivity to small molecule TKIs has been found. This may be because expression of EGFR at the cell surface does not take into account the decreased or increased activity of a mutant receptor, whether the receptor is internalized to the nucleus, whether the signaling pathway downstream of EGFR is active, or a combination of these factors. Moreover, the presence of EGFR does not imply that the tumor cell is dependent on this signal pathway for growth or survival, because many alternative mitogenic signaling pathways are available to tumor cells [51,55].

Preclinical studies performed on bladder cancer cell lines indicate that gefitinib affects many of the same intracellular signaling pathways inhibited by anti-EGFR mAb therapy [64–66]. Gefitinib inhibits the growth of a range of human bladder TCC cell lines in vitro by inducing cell-cycle arrest, apoptosis, or both [67–69]. The antitumor effect and potentiation of cytotoxic drugs in human cancer cells by TKIs are now well documented, and provide a good basis for its use in clinically advanced bladder cancer as adjuncts to systemic chemotherapy for muscle-invasive bladder cancer [70].

As described so far, the erbB family represents one of the many potential targets against TCC of the bladder. Antiangiogenic therapy is another targeted pathway that holds potential in urothelial carcinoma. An increasing number of drugs are being developed against angiogenesis. Animal studies using different antiangiogenesis strategies have demonstrated the ability to limit TCC growth. Strategies have included the use of antibodies targeting specific inducers, such as VEGF [71].

VEGF is an extensively studied inducer of angiogenesis. As a prognostic marker in bladder cancer, higher levels of VEGF in tumor tissue predict an increased risk of progression of T1 disease, and elevated urinary levels are a marker of increased risk of recurrence for patients with superficial lesions [71]. Recently, overexpression of VEGF in prechemotherapy samples from patients with locally advanced urothelial cancer who were undergoing cystectomy and chemotherapy was found to be a strong predictor of recurrence and death from bladder cancer [72]. This observation presents the important hypothesis that VEGF expression is mechanistically relevant to clinically aggressive bladder cancer and provides rationale for the clinical investigation of interventions capable of blocking VEGF signaling. Multiple agents are under investigation in phase I to III studies; specific indications for bladder cancer await future trials.

Future approaches for targeted therapy: the algorithm concept?

The tremendous amount of data accumulated through genomics, proteomics, and metabolomic technologies has not led to a definitive understanding of the mechanisms underlying cancer. The challenge remains as to how to integrate all of the relevant knowledge and data in a systematic manner so that researchers can gain the knowledge needed to devise the best therapeutic and diagnostic strategies. Human TCC of the bladder is genetically heterogeneous, and it is surrounded by a complex tissue microenvironment involving vasculature, stromal cells, and connective tissue. One of the most challenging problems facing cancer researchers is the lack of correlation between in vitro cell lines and animal tumor models and human in vivo tumors. A few promising approaches are being devised that will help address this issue in the coming years [73]. One such approach is the measurement of molecular levels of receptors, ligands, pathways components, and so on, directly in human tumors through in vivo imaging [74], or through proteomic profiling,

as it has been proposed as standard protocol for cancer diagnostics and therapeutics [75–77].

Another approach might involve the use of improved in vitro systems to better mimic human in vivo tumors. The correlation of in vitro systems, which are more prone to experimental perturbations for uncovering disease mechanisms or therapeutic strategies, with in vivo systems and vice versa represents an important approach for studying human TCC of the bladder. Thus, a range of different bladder carcinoma cell lines could be used as a basis for creating an in vivo model based on molecular data collected from humans. The in vivo models could then be used to directly predict the efficacy of a given therapy in patients and to consequently characterize the molecular biomarkers that can predict efficacy and toxicity. Thus, one can envision a scenario in which, based on accumulated data, the urologist can create a complex algorithm that will identify the best therapy for a subgroup of patients who "fit" a known biologic pattern. The road map for developing such a system will require linking experimental data to computational approaches that can simulate known biologic systems, also known as system biology [78,79], that can potentially revolutionize our understanding of bladder cancer.

References

[1] Jemal A, Tiwari RC, Murray T, et al. Cancer statistics, 2004. CA Cancer J Clin 2004;54:8–29.
[2] Geller NL, Sternberg CN, Penenberg D, et al. Prognostic factors for survival of patients with advanced urothelial tumors treated with methotrexate, vinblastine, doxorubicin, and cisplatin chemotherapy. Cancer 1991;67:1525–31.
[3] Sternberg CN, Yagoda A, Scher HI, et al. W.F. M-VAC (methotrexate, vinblastine, doxorubicin and cisplatin) for advanced transitional cell carcinoma of the urothelium. J Urol 1988;139:461–9.
[4] Logothetis CJ, Finn LD, Smith T, et al. Escalated MVAC with or without recombinant human granulocyte-macrophage colony-stimulating factor for initial treatment of advanced malignant urothelial tumors: results of a randomized trial. J Clin Oncol 1995;13:2272–7.
[5] Roth BJ, Dreicer R, Einhorn LH, et al. Significant activity of paclitaxel in advanced transitional cell carcinoma of the urothelium: a phase II trial of the Eastern Cooperative Oncology Group. J Clin Oncol 1994;12:2264–70.
[6] Vaughn DJ, Malkowicz SB, Zoltick B, et al. Paclitaxel plus carboplatin in advanced carcinoma of

the urothelium: an active and tolerable outpatient regimen. J Clin Oncol 1998;16:255–60.

[7] Redman BG, Smith DC, Flaherty L, et al. Phase II trial of paclitaxel and carboplatin in the treatment of advanced urothelial carcinoma. J Clin Oncol 1998;16:1844–8.

[8] Bajorin DF, McCafrey JA, Hilton S, et al. Treatment of patients with transitional-cell carcinoma of the urothelial tract with ifosfamide, paclitaxel, and cisplatin: a phase II trial. J Clin Oncol 1998;16:2722–7.

[9] Von der Maase H, Hansen SW, Roberts JT, et al. Gemcitabine and cisplatin versus methotrexate, vinblastine, doxorubicin, and cisplatin in advanced or metastatic bladder cancer: results of a large randomized, multinational, multicenter, phase III study. J Clin Oncol 2000;17:3068–77.

[10] Hussain M, Vaishampayan U, Du W, et al. Combination carboplatin, paclitaxel and gemcitabine. Is an active teatment for advanced urothelial carcinoma. J Clin Oncol 2001;19:2527–33.

[11] Cote RJ, Datar RH. Therapeutic approaches to bladder cancer: identifying targets and mechanisms. Crit Rev Oncol Hematol 2003;46(Suppl):S67–83.

[12] Ullrich A, Coussens L, Hayflick JS, et al. Human epidermal growth factor receptor cDNA sequence and aberrant expression of the amplified gene in A431 epidermoid carcinoma cells. Nature 1984; 309(5967):418–25.

[13] Gullick WJ. The Type 1 growth factor receptors and their ligands considered as a complex system. Endocr Relat Cancer 2001;8(2):75–82.

[14] Salomon DS, Normanno N, Ciardiello F, et al. The role of amphiregulin in breast cancer. Breast Cancer Res Treat 1995;33(2):103–14.

[15] Yarden Y. Biology of HER2 and its importance in breast cancer. Oncology 2001;61(Suppl 2):1–13.

[16] Nicholson RI, Gee JM, Harper ME. EGFR and cancer prognosis. Eur J Cancer 2001;37(Suppl 4): S9–15.

[17] Mendelsohn J. The epidermal growth factor receptor as a target for cancer therapy. Endocr Relat Cancer 2001;8(1):3–9.

[18] Neal DE, Mellon K. Epidermal growth factor receptor and bladder cancer: a review. Urol Int 1992; 48(4):365–71.

[19] Lipponen P, Eskelinen M. Expression of epidermal growth factor receptor in bladder cancer as related to established prognostic factors, oncoprotein (c-erbB-2, p53) expression and long-term prognosis. Br J Cancer 1994;69(6):1120–5.

[20] Sauter G, Maeda T, Waldman FM, et al. Patterns of epidermal growth factor receptor amplification in malignant gliomas. Am J Pathol 1996;148(4): 1047–53.

[21] Turkeri LN, Erton ML, Cevik I, Akdas A. Impact of the expression of epidermal growth factor, transforming growth factor alpha, and epidermal growth factor receptor on the prognosis of superficial bladder cancer. Urology 1998;51(4):645–9.

[22] Neal DE, Sharples L, Smith K, et al. The epidermal growth factor receptor and the prognosis of bladder cancer. Cancer 1990;65(7):1619–25.

[23] Chow NH, Chan SH, Tzai TS, et al. Expression profiles of erbB family receptors and prognosis in primary transitional cell carcinoma of the urinary bladder. Clin Cancer Res 2001;7(7):1957–62.

[24] Nguyen PL, Swanson PE, Jaszcz W, et al. Expression of epidermal growth factor receptor in invasive transitional cell carcinoma of the urinary bladder. A multivariate survival analysis. Am J Clin Pathol 1994;101(2):166–76.

[25] Messing EM. Clinical implications of the expression of epidermal growth factor receptors in human transitional cell carcinoma. Cancer Res 1990;50(8): 2530–7.

[26] Popov Z, Gil-Diez-De-Medina S, Ravery V, et al. Prognostic value of EGF receptor and tumor cell proliferation in bladder cancer: therapeutic implications. Urol Oncol 2004;22(2):93–101.

[27] Chow NH, Liu HS, Yang HB, et al. Expression patterns of erbB receptor family in normal urothelium and transitional cell carcinoma. An immunohistochemical study. Virchows Arch 1997;430(6): 461–6.

[28] Rajkumar T, Gullick WJ. The type I growth factor receptors in human breast cancer. Breast Cancer Res Treat 1994;29(1):3–9.

[29] Sriplakich S, Jahnson S, Karlsson MG. Epidermal growth factor receptor expression: predictive value for the outcome after cystectomy for bladder cancer? BJU Int 1999;83(4):498–503.

[30] Jimenez RE, Hussain M, Bianco FJ Jr, et al. Her-2/neu overexpression in muscle-invasive urothelial carcinoma of the bladder: prognostic significance and comparative analysis in primary and metastatic tumors. Clin Cancer Res 2001;7(8):2440–7.

[31] Lonn U, Lonn S, Friberg S, Nilsson B, et al. Prognostic value of amplification of c-erb-B2 in bladder carcinoma. Clin Cancer Res 1995;1(10):1189–94.

[32] Liukkonen T, Rajala P, Raitanen M, et al. Prognostic value of MIB-1 score, p53, EGFr, mitotic index and papillary status in primary superficial (Stage pTa/T1) bladder cancer: a prospective comparative study. The Finnbladder Group. Eur Urol 1999; 36(5):393–400.

[33] Kruger S, Weitsch G, Buttner H, et al. HER2 overexpression in muscle-invasive urothelial carcinoma of the bladder: prognostic implications. Int J Cancer 2002;102(5):514–8.

[34] Gandour-Edwards R, Lara PN Jr, Folkins AK, et al. Does HER2/neu expression provide prognostic information in patients with advanced urothelial carcinoma? Cancer 2002;95(5):1009–15.

[35] Junttila TT, Laato M, Vahlberg T, et al. Identification of patients with transitional cell carcinoma of the bladder overexpressing erbB2, erbB3, or specific erbB4 isoforms: real-time reverse transcription-PCR analysis in estimation of erbB receptor

status from cancer patients. Clin Cancer Res 2003; 9(14):5346–57.

[36] Lynch TJ, Bell DW, Sordella R, et al. Activating mutations in the epidermal growth factor receptor underlying responsiveness of non-small-cell lung cancer to gefitinib. N Engl J Med 2004;350(21): 2129–39 (Epub 2004 Apr 29).

[37] Paez JG, Janne PA, Lee JC, et al. EGFR mutations in lung cancer: correlation with clinical response to gefitinib therapy. Science 2004;304(5676):1497–500 (Epub 2004 Apr 29).

[38] Barber TD, Vogelstein B, Kinzler KW, et al. Somatic mutations of EGFR in colorectal cancers and glioblastomas. N Engl J Med 2004;351(27): 2883.

[39] Sordella R, Bell DW, Haber DA, et al. Gefitinib-sensitizing EGFR mutations in lung cancer activate anti-apoptotic pathways. Science 2004;305(5687): 1163–7 (Epub 2004 Jul 29).

[40] Zhan Y, O'Rourke DM. SHP-2-dependent mitogen-activated protein kinase activation regulates EGFR-vIII but not wild-type epidermal growth factor receptor phosphorylation and glioblastoma cell survival. Cancer Res 2004;64(22):8292–8.

[41] Learn CA, Hartzell TL, Wikstrand CJ, et al. Resistance to tyrosine kinase inhibition by mutant epidermal growth factor receptor variant III contributes to the neoplastic phenotype of glioblastoma multiforme. Clin Cancer Res 2004;10(9):3216–24.

[42] David M, Wong L, Flavell R, et al. STAT activation by epidermal growth factor (EGF) and amphiregulin. Requirement for the EGF receptor kinase but not for tyrosine phosphorylation sites or JAK1. J Biol Chem 1996;271(16):9185–8.

[43] Lin SY, Makino K, Xia W, et al. Nuclear localization of EGF receptor and its potential new role as a transcription factor. Nat Cell Biol 2001;3(9):802–8.

[44] Bargmann CI, Hung MC, Weinberg RA. The neu oncogene encodes an epidermal growth factor receptor-related protein. Nature 1986;319(6050):226–30.

[45] Longo N, Shuster RC, Griffin LD, et al. Activation of insulin receptor signaling by a single amino acid substitution in the transmembrane domain. J Biol Chem 1992;267(18):12416–9.

[46] Williams CC, Allison JG, Vidal GA, et al. The ERBB4/HER4 receptor tyrosine kinase regulates gene expression by functioning as a STAT5A nuclear chaperone. J Cell Biol 2004;167(3):469–78.

[47] Swindle CS, Tran KT, Johnson TD, et al. Epidermal growth factor (EGF)-like repeats of human tenascin-C as ligands for EGF receptor. J Cell Biol 2001;154(2):459–68.

[48] Adam RM, Eaton SH, Estrada C, et al. Mechanical stretch is a highly selective regulator of gene expression in human bladder smooth muscle cells. Physiol Genomics 2004;20(1):36–44 (Epub 2004 Oct 5).

[49] Gill GN, Bertics PJ, Santon JB. Epidermal growth factor and its receptor. Mol Cell Endocrinol 1987; 51(3):169–86.

[50] Zwick E, Hackel PO, Prenzel N, et al. The EGF receptor as central transducer of heterologous signalling systems. Trends Pharmacol Sci 1999;20(10): 408–12.

[51] Prenzel N, Zwick E, Leserer M, et al. Tyrosine kinase signalling in breast cancer. Epidermal growth factor receptor: convergence point for signal integration and diversification. Breast Cancer Res 2000; 2(3):184–90 (Epub 2000 Mar 25).

[52] Uchiyama-Tanaka Y, Matsubara H, Nozawa Y, et al. Angiotensin II signaling and HB-EGF shedding via metalloproteinase in glomerular mesangial cells. Kidney Int 2001;60(6):2153–63.

[53] McCole DF, Keely SJ, Coffey RJ, et al. Transactivation of the epidermal growth factor receptor in colonic epithelial cells by carbachol requires extracellular release of transforming growth factor-alpha. J Biol Chem 2002;277(45):42603–12 (Epub 2002 Aug 28).

[54] Schafer B, Marg B, Gschwind A, et al. Distinct ADAM metalloproteinases regulate G protein-coupled receptor-induced cell proliferation and survival. J Biol Chem 2004;279(46):47929–38 (Epub 2004 Aug 26).

[55] Gschwind A, Zwick E, Prenzel N, et al. Cell communication networks: epidermal growth factor receptor transactivation as the paradigm for interreceptor signal transmission. Oncogene 2001;20(13): 1594–600.

[56] Slamon DJ, Leyland-Jones B, Shak S, et al. Use of chemotherapy plus a monoclonal antibody against HER2 for metastatic breast cancer that overexpress HER2. N Engl J Med 2001;344:783–92.

[57] Cobleigh MA, Vogel CL, Tripathy D, et al. Multinational study of the efficacy and safety of humanized anti-HER2 monoclonal antibody in women who have HER2-overexpressing metastatic breast cancer that has progressed after chemotherapy for metastatic disease. J Clin Oncol 1999;17: 2639–48.

[58] Miller VA, Johnson D, Heelan RT, et al. A pilot trial demonstrates the safety of ZD1839 (Iressa), an oral epidermal growth factor receptor tyrosine kinase inhibitor (EGFR-TKI), in combination with carboplatin and paclitaxel in previously untreated advanced non-small cell lung cancer. J Clin Oncol 2003;21(11):2094–100.

[59] Giaccone G, Herbst RS, Manegold C, et al. Gefitinib in combination with gemcitabine and cisplatin in advanced non-small-cell lung cancer: a phase III trial–INTACT 1. J Clin Oncol 2004;22:777–84.

[60] Herbst RS, Giaccone G, Schiller JH, et al. Gefitinib in combination with paclitaxel and carboplatin in advanced non-small-cell lung cancer: a phase III trial–INTACT 2. J Clin Oncol 2004;22:785–94.

[61] Moulder SL, Yakes FM, Muthuswamy SK, et al. Epidermal growth factor receptor (HER1) tyrosine kinase inhibitor ZD1839 (Iressa) inhibits HER2/neu (erbB2)-overexpressing breast cancer cells

in vitro and in vivo. Cancer Res 2001;61(24): 8887–95.

[62] Bishop PC, Myers T, Robey R, et al. Differential sensitivity of cancer cells to inhibitors of the epidermal growth factor receptor family. Oncogene 2002; 21(1):119–27.

[63] Harari PM. Epidermal growth factor receptor inhibition strategies in oncology. Endocr Relat Cancer 2004;11(4):689–708.

[64] Ennis BW, Lippman ME, Dickson RB. The EGF receptor system as a target for antitumor therapy. Cancer Invest 1991;9(5):553–62.

[65] Inoue K, Slaton JW, Davis DW, et al. Treatment of human metastatic transitional cell carcinoma of the bladder in a murine model with the anti-vascular endothelial growth factor receptor monoclonal antibody DC101 and paclitaxel. Clin Cancer Res 2000; 6:2635–43.

[66] Woodburn JR. The epidermal growth factor receptor and its inhibition in cancer therapy. Pharmacol Ther 1999;82(2–3):241–50.

[67] Perrotte P, Matsumoto T, Inoue K, et al. Anti-epidermal growth factor receptor antibody C225 inhibits angiogenesis in human transitional cell carcinoma growing orthotopically in nude mice. Clin Cancer Res 1999;5(2):257–65.

[68] Maddineni SB, Sangar VK, Hendry JH, et al. Differential radiosensitisation by ZD1839 (Iressa), a highly selective epidermal growth factor receptor tyrosine kinase inhibitor in two related bladder cancer cell lines. Br J Cancer 2005;92(1):125–30.

[69] Nutt JE, Lazarowicz HP, Mellon JK, et al. Gefitinib ("Iressa," ZD1839) inhibits the growth response of bladder tumour cell lines to epidermal growth factor and induces TIMP2. Br J Cancer 2004;90(8): 1679–85.

[70] McHugh LA, Griffiths TR, Kriajevska M, et al. Tyrosine kinase inhibitors of the epidermal growth factor receptor as adjuncts to systemic chemotherapy for muscle-invasive bladder cancer. Urology 2004;63(4):619–24.

[71] Crew JP. Vascular endothelial growth factor: an important angiogenic mediator in bladder cancer. Eur Urol 1999;35:2.

[72] Slaton JW, Millikan R, Inoue K, et al. Correlation of metastasis related gene expression and relapse-free survival in patients with locally advanced bladder cancer treated with cystectomy and chemotherapy. J Urol 2001;171:570.

[73] Khalil IG, Hill C. Systems biology for cancer. Curr Opin Oncol 2005;17(1):44–8.

[74] Chen G, Gharib TG, Wang H, et al. Protein profiles associated with survival in lung adenocarcinoma. Proc Natl Acad Sci USA 2003;100(23):13537–42 (Epub 2003 Oct 22).

[75] Petricoin EF, Ornstein DK, Liotta LA. Clinical proteomics: applications for prostate cancer biomarker discovery and detection. Urol Oncol 2004;22(4): 322–8.

[76] Baggerly KA, Deng L, Morris JS, et al. Overdispersed logistic regression for SAGE: modelling multiple groups and covariates. BMC Bioinformatics 2004;5(1):144.

[77] Geho DH, Petricoin EF, Liotta LA. Blasting into the microworld of tissue proteomics: a new window on cancer. Clin Cancer Res 2004;10(3):825–7.

[78] Hendriks BS, Opresko LK, Wiley HS, et al. Quantitative analysis of HER2-mediated effects on HER2 and epidermal growth factor receptor endocytosis: distribution of homo- and heterodimers depends on relative HER2 levels. J Biol Chem 2003;278(26): 23343–51 (Epub 2003 Apr 9).

[79] Resat H, Ewald JA, Dixon DA, et al. An integrated model of epidermal growth factor receptor trafficking and signal transduction. Biophys J 2003;85(2): 730–43.

ELSEVIER
SAUNDERS

Urol Clin N Am 32 (2005) 247–252

UROLOGIC
CLINICS
of North America

Index

Note: Page numbers of article titles are in **boldface** type.

Changing Your Address?

Make sure your subscription changes too! When you notify us of your new address, you can help make our job easier by including an exact copy of your Clinics label number with your old address (see illustration below.) This number identifies you to our computer system and will speed the processing of your address change. Please be sure this label number accompanies your old address and your corrected address—you can send an old Clinics label with your number on it or just copy it exactly and send it to the address listed below.

We appreciate your help in our attempt to give you continuous coverage. Thank you.

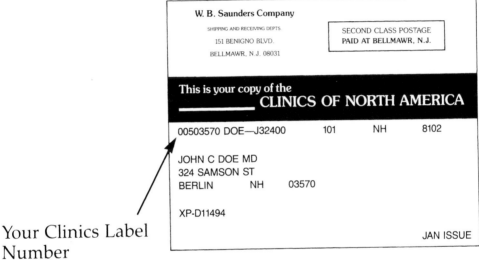

W. B. Saunders Company

SHIPPING AND RECEIVING DEPTS
151 BENIGNO BLVD.
BELLMAWR, N.J. 08031

SECOND CLASS POSTAGE
PAID AT BELLMAWR, N.J.

This is your copy of the
CLINICS OF NORTH AMERICA

00503570 DOE—J32400   101   NH   8102

JOHN C DOE MD
324 SAMSON ST
BERLIN   NH   03570

XP-D11494

JAN ISSUE

Your Clinics Label Number
Copy it exactly or send your label
along with your address to:
W.B. Saunders Company, Customer Service
Orlando, FL 32887-4800
Call Toll Free 1-800-654-2452

Please allow four to six weeks for delivery of new subscriptions and for processing address changes.